1981

HEALTH CARE
AND THE ELDERLY

C. Carl Pegels
State University of New York at Buffalo

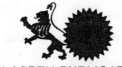

AN ASPEN PUBLICATION®
Aspen Systems Corporation
Rockville, Maryland
London
1980

Library of Congress Cataloging in Publication Data

Pegels, C. Carl.
Health care and the elderly.

Includes bibliographical references and index.

1. Aged—Medical care—United States. 2. Aged—
Care and hygiene—United States. I. Title.
[DNLM: 1. Delivery of health care—United States.
2. Aged. 3. Geriatrics—United States. WT30 P376h]
RA564.8.P43   362.1'9897'00973   80-24360
ISBN: 0-89443-333-4

Library of Congress Catalog Card Number: 80-24360
ISBN: 0-89443-333-4

Printed in the United States of America

1 2 3 4 5

Table of Contents

Preface

This book has evolved over a relatively long time. The initial impetus for it arose from an interest in and a concern for the nursing home patient during the early- to mid-seventies. Nursing home patients and the nursing home controversy were prominent topics for discussion in those days.

Since then concern about health care for all of the elderly has become more prominent. Although nursing homes consume an inordinate amount of the health care dollar allotted for the elderly population, only about 5 percent of the elderly actually reside in them. The health care of the other 95 percent is equally important. Therefore, this book attempts to deal with the entire domain of health care for the elderly, devoting approximately equal attention to nursing-home-based health care and nonnursing-home-based health care, including home care, day care, ambulatory care, vision and hearing care, drug therapy, and dental care.

People connected with specific aspects of health care delivery as it applies to the elderly may not always agree with the views presented or the conclusions drawn in many chapters. This book, however, is intended to provide an unbiased overview of current and prospective health care delivery to the elderly.

Well-intentioned government officials at the federal, state, and local levels, as well as health care practitioners, will quite understandably resent the critical and sometimes pessimistic views presented in certain chapters. However, problem areas must be identified before corrective action can be taken. As compensation for many of the critical, pessimistic, or negative views there are numerous positive aspects to the health and health care of the elderly. Most elderly people are healthy and live vigorous and happy lives with minimal need of health care; health care may not be an important topic to such people. They should, however, share responsibility for and be instrumental in alleviating the numerous problems still unresolved in today's health care for the elderly.

This book is oriented toward facts and issues. The facts consist largely of statistical data obtained from many sources, especially government sources. As much as possible, credit has been given to all sources of data and information.

Several graduate students helped me with the data and information collection. Without their support this book would not have been written. Therefore, I want to give credit and thanks, in alphabetical order, to Michael Choo, Jeffrey Forster, Steven Gabor, Paul Gworek, Peter Margulis, Kyle McNeil and Harry Schultz, all one-time graduate students in the School of Management and in the Center for Policy Studies at the State University of New York at Buffalo.

I want to thank also the authors of Chapters 14 and 21 for allowing me to use their previously published journal articles in this book. Without secretarial support this book would not have been completed. Many thanks to all the secretaries who worked on the manuscript at one time or another, and special thanks to Marilyn Viau who worked on the later drafts.

C. Carl Pegels
December 1980

Chapter 1

The Present and Future of Health Care for the Aged

T he aged, those Americans age 65 and over, presently comprise about 11 percent of the United States population. Fifty years from now this figure is expected to increase to an estimated 17 to 20 percent. This increase is not entirely due to increased longevity; it also reflects the post-World War II baby boom and the present lowered birthrate. It is assumed that for the foreseeable future the birthrate will continue to be depressed.

Since the aged are disproportionately high utilizers of health care, and since over two-thirds of all health care costs for the aged are paid for with public funds, it is not surprising that there is considerable interest in projected population figures for the aged.

This introductory chapter presents some demographics that describe the present and future aged population and determines the financial impact of a near doubling of the aged population percentage. The chapter concludes with a brief overview of topics covered in the balance of the book.

POPULATION DEMOGRAPHICS—PAST AND PRESENT

In the 70 years between 1900 and 1970, the total U.S. population almost tripled. The segment comprising those people age 65 and over grew to almost seven times its size in 1900. This segment is still growing faster than the under-65 population segment. Between 1960 and 1970, the group of Americans 65 and over increased by 21 percent, as compared with a 13 percent population increase for the under-65 group.

During 1960-70 the percentages increased most dramatically in Arizona, Florida, Nevada, Hawaii, and New Mexico. In each of these states the population 65 and over increased by at least one-third. These five states plus Alaska were the fastest growing in 1970-75 as well. Florida, which experienced a considerable influx of older persons, had the highest *proportion* of older people— 14.5 percent in 1970 and 16.1 percent in 1975. In 1975 California became the state with the largest *number* of older people—2,056,000—outnumbering New York which was first in 1970 with 2,030,000 elderly.

As a group, the older population is neither homogeneous nor static. Every day approximately five thousand Americans reach age 65, and approximately thirty-six hundred persons age 65 and over die. This yields a net increase in the aged population—about fourteen hundred per day, or half a million per year.

POPULATION DEMOGRAPHICS—PRESENT AND FUTURE

The 1980 population of about 222 million Americans consists of 198 million people (89.2 percent) under 65 and 24 million people (10.8 percent) age 65 and over. The 24 million elderly include about 9.3 million people over 75 years of age. Because of increased longevity, the number of elderly over 75 years of age is expected to grow even more rapidly than the number of elderly between 65 and 75. In fact, the population 75 years and older is projected to grow from 9.3 million in 1980 to 12.4 million in the year 2000. By 2030 this group is expected to number about 25 million.

Table 1-1 summarizes this population data and lists the sources from which most of the data is taken. Some of the data represents extrapolations by the author. Making population projections is a rather hazardous venture. Even a minor change in assumptions can result in dramatic differences in numbers, espe-

Table 1-1 Demographic Projections of U.S. Population

Source	Year	Total Population (in millions)	Population 65+	Population 75+
AHCA[1]	1980	222	24.0 (10.8%)	9.3 (4.2%)
AHCA[1]	1990	239	27.6 (11.5%)	11.0 (4.6%)
AHCA[1]	2000	251	28.3 (11.3%)	12.4 (4.9%)
Bureau of Census[4]	2000	251	31.0 (12.4%)	—
Panneton and Wesolowski[3]	2000	251	33.0 (13.1%)	13.3 (5.3%)
Panneton and Wesolowski[3]	2030	280	56.0 (20.0%)	28.0 (10.0%)
Kovar[2]	2030	280	51.0 (18.2%)	25.5 (9.1%)
Bureau of Census[4]	2030	271	46.0 (17.0%)	25.0 (9.2%)

Sources: 1. American Health Care Association (AHCA), "Long Term Care Facts" (Chicago: AHCA, 1975).

2. M. G. Kovar, "Health of the Elderly and Use of Health Services," *Public Health Reports* 92 (January-February 1977): 9-19.

3. P. E. Panneton and E. F. Wesolowski, "Current and Future Needs in Geriatric Education," *Public Health Reports* 94 (January-February 1979): 73-79.

4. U.S. Bureau of the Census, Publications relating to population and health statistics.

cially when one projects as far as 50 years into the future. The only consolation is that one can be proven wrong only 50 years from now.

HEALTH STATUS OF OLDER PEOPLE

If we assume that average life expectancy will increase over the next 20 years, and that this increase will come not from a slowing of the rate of aging, but from continuingly improved health, it follows that we are also assuming improved health status for future generations of older persons.

In truth, the realities are more complex. The relationships of various forms of morbidity to mortality are not well understood. Both morbidity and mortality are affected by educational level and socioeconomic status. Nor do we completely understand the relationships between mortality rates at younger ages and mortality rates at later ages. Furthermore, "health" or "vigor" can be defined and measured in various ways. It suffices to say that in the future older persons will experience improved levels of health because poverty is diminishing over the life cycles of successive generations, because educational levels are rising, and because there will be more effective forms of public health and improved systems of health care.

QUANTITY VERSUS QUALITY OF LIFE

From a demographic point of view, progress in the "control" or management of the aging process is measured principally in terms of an increase in the "quantity" of life. This means, for example, reductions in mortality rates and increases in survival rates or in average life expectancies. But progress can also be measured in terms of improvements in the "quality" of life—that is, by reducing the incidence and prevalence rates for morbidity, mental illness, and disability. Life quality can also be measured in terms of the proportions of elderly hospitalized and institutionalized, and the proportions of widowed or living alone. A principal goal of public and private effort should be to make the later years of life vigorous, healthy, and satisfying, instead of merely adding years to life.

PROSPECTS FOR MORTALITY REDUCTION

The future number of elderly persons is directly dependent on the progress made in reducing death rates at the older ages and at the younger ages. Some reductions could be achieved by earlier diagnosis and treatment of major illnesses and by mass screening and follow-up.

Death is often the result of multiple causes; even if one cause is eliminated, the other causes may still lead to death, although possibly with some time lag. Moreover, if deaths from a particular cause (say, cancer) were eliminated or sharply reduced, those people saved would be subject to death from other causes (for example, heart disease). Conceivably, the mortality rates from these other causes could result in a rise in the general death rate.

HEALTH NEEDS OF THE ELDERLY

Health care and retirement income are probably the most critical issues affecting the well-being of senior citizens. For individuals who face problems of both health and income, the problems often have a ruinous compound impact. The health and income of older Americans are so highly interrelated, especially for the elderly poor, that the situation resembles the classic "chicken or egg" quandary. Does low income bring on poor health, or does poor health bring on low income?

A quick review of the economic status of older people shows that about 3.3 million are below the poverty line, with an additional 2.2 million "near poor." The two groups combined represent more than one-quarter of all the elderly. In many instances poverty is the result of loss of earned income at retirement. It is interesting to note that, on the average, older couples receive less than half the income of younger couples.

In contrast to the younger family's budget, the typical retired couple's budget is dominated by essential items and includes very little money for discretionary spending. Figures from the Bureau of Labor Statistics (BLS) show that older consumers spend a greater share of their income for food, shelter, medical care, and transportation than do their younger counterparts. According to BLS, a full 80 percent of the intermediate level retired couple's budget is eaten up by these four basic expenses.

Of particular note is the fact that medical care prices have consistently increased faster than the general cost of living, especially during the last ten years. This increase has been matched by an increase in the percent of gross national product spent for health care.

Although older people comprise just 11 percent of the total population, they account for 29 percent of the national expenditures for personal health care. As the major consumers of health services, the elderly have a vital interest in cost and quality controls and in service improvements.

Contrary to popular thinking, Medicare, Medicaid, and the other health programs have not resolved the health cost problems of older people. Despite these public programs, and despite private health insurance coverage, the elderly must still pay 30 percent of their personal health care bills out of pocket.

Since the institution of Medicare, the bulk of the increase in older persons' private health care expenses has covered the two major gaps in Medicare coverage—long-term care and outpatient prescription drugs. Although Medicare protection does cover a major portion of hospital and physician services, the individual's financial burden is unreasonably large and needs to be further insured.

Chronic and acute disabling conditions pose special health problems for the elderly. In social terms, chronic disabling conditions pose extra problems because they directly affect the self-maintenance capacities of older people. The loss or impairment of the ability to perform such basic daily functions as shopping or bathing strikes at what the elderly value most—independent living.

Because only five percent of the present aged population are institutionalized, there is an unfortunate tendency to minimize the importance of nursing homes when analyzing the health delivery system. The role of nursing homes has been put into a more accurate perspective with the finding that 20 percent of the older population will, sooner or later, spend some time in a nursing home.

Older people also have more problems with mental illness than does the general population. Among adults age 25 and over, those over 65 are at least twice as likely to be hospitalized for mental conditions than those under 65. The suicide rate provides another index of mental problems. The rate increases with age, is higher for men than for women, and peaks among older men.

HEALTH CARE EXPENDITURES

The Present

The entire U.S. population spent $120.5 billion for personal health care during the 1976 Federal fiscal year.[5] Of this total, about $34.9 billion (29 percent) was spent on health care for those age 65 years and older; the remaining $85.6 billion (71 percent) was spent on health care for those under 65.

Based on a population base of about 215 million people—including 22.9 million (10.65 percent) elderly—the per capita personal health care expenditure for the elderly amounted to $1,524. This compares to a per capita personal health care expenditure of $446 for those under 65. In other words, the cost of personal health care for those age 65 and over is about 3.4 times greater than the cost for those under 65. Table 1-2 itemizes these statistics in detail.

The Future

Table 1-3 shows present health care expenditures projected to the year 2030. These costs are shown in terms of 1976 dollars to obtain a useful comparison.

The population in 2030 is projected at 280 million, consisting of 51 million (18.2 percent) people age 65 and older, and 229 million people under 65. Per capita health care expenditures are projected to remain unchanged—that is, $1,524 for those 65 years and over and $446 for those under 65.

Table 1-2 Health Care Expenditures—1976

	Population 65−	Population 65+	Total Population
Personal Health Care Dollars	$85.6B	$34.9B	$120.5B
Personal Health Care Percent	71%	29%	100%
Population Percent	89.35%	10.65%	100%
Population Numbers	192.1M	22.9M	215M
Per Capita Expenditures	$446	$1,524	$560
Ratio to 65- Population	1.0	3.41	1.26

Sources: National Center for Health Statistics, *Health, U.S.* (Washington, D.C.: U.S. Government Printing Office, 1978).

U.S. Bureau of the Census, *Statistical Abstracts of U.S.* (Washington, D.C.: U.S. Government Printing Office, 1978).

The increase in population means that total personal health care expenditures will increase to $102.1 billion for those under 65 and to $77.6 billion for those age 65 and over. The total annual dollar expenditure in 2030 will reach $179.7 billion, an increase of $59.2 billion over the 1976 figure.

Adjusting the 2030 health care expenditures for the increase in population from 215 million to 280 million results in an annual personal health care expenditure of $138 billion in 2030. The $17.5 billion increase (14.5 percent)

Table 1-3 Health Care Expenditures—2030 (in 1976 Dollars)

	Population 65−	Population 65+	Total Population
Population Numbers	229M	51M	280M
Population Percent	71.8%	18.2%	100%
Per Capita Expenditures	$446	$1,524	$642
Personal Health Care Dollars	$102.1B	$77.6B	$179.7B
Personal Health Care Percent	57%	43%	100%

Note: Total personal health care expenditures increased from $120.5 billion to $179.7 billion, an increase of 49.1%. However, total population also increased from 215 million to 280 million, an increase of 30.2%. Hence, the adjusted total personal health care expenditures in 2030 is 215/280 ($179.7 billion) or $138.0 billion, which represents only a 14.5% increase.

Sources: National Center for Health Statistics, *Health, U.S.,* (Washington, D.C.: U.S. Government Printing Office, 1978).

U.S. Bureau of Census, *Statistical Abstracts of U.S.,* (Washington, D.C.: U.S. Government Printing Office, 1978).

over the 1976 figure is due entirely to the increase in the elderly population—from 10.65 percent to a projected 18.2 percent.

This analysis shows that 50 years from now the total cost of personal health care will increase by only 14.5 percent, due to the increase of the elderly population from 10.65 percent to a projected 18.2 percent. It is assumed, of course, that everything else will remain unchanged. The critical point is that the country's total personal health care bill will continue to rise but that this increase cannot be blamed on the elderly. The analysis shows clearly that the increase in the number of elderly affects total health care costs by only 14.5 percent.

HOW THIS BOOK IS ORGANIZED

This book is organized in three parts. Part 1 covers such topics as the historical development of long-term health care; an analysis of the effects of costs, expenditures, and inflation on health care; an analysis of information, referral, and support services; and cost benefit alternatives in health care. This section concludes with a discussion of home health care, day health care, and assessment and placement of the non-well elderly.

Part 2 covers institutionalization of the non-well elderly in the nursing home. Chapters cover such topics as the nursing home industry, the nursing home and its residents, dimensions of the nursing home controversy, medical direction in skilled nursing homes, the physician extender in the nursing home, legal perspectives of nursing homes, and reorganization of the nursing home industry.

Part 3 is devoted to special topics such as vision, hearing, and dental care; development of a national health policy; supplementary health insurance and prepaid care; quality of care versus reduction in costs; health manpower issues; terminal care and the hospice; and the future of health care for the elderly.

CONCLUSIONS

This first chapter has provided a setting for the important topic of health care for the elderly. The elderly are never explicitly blamed for the rapid expansion of health care costs. But the fact that the cost of providing personal health care to the elderly is nearly 3.5 times the cost of providing personal health care to the balance of the population may create the impression that the elderly are responsible.

Older people are more likely to be afflicted with one or more ailments. Since accessible health care is increasingly considered a right instead of a privilege, it is fitting that society at large should bear the burden of providing the resources that ensure personal health care for those afflicted.

In the balance of this book we shall present, discuss, and analyze the various dimensions of providing health care to the elderly.

NOTES

1. American Health Care Association (AHCA), "Long Term Care Facts" (Chicago: AHCA, 1975).
2. M. G. Kovar, "Health of the Elderly and Use of Health Services," *Public Health Reports* 92 (January-February 1977): 9-19.
3. P. E. Panneton and E. F. Wesolowski, "Current and Future Needs in Geriatric Education," *Public Health Reports* 94 (January-February 1979): 73-79.
4. U.S. Bureau of the Census, Publications relating to population and health statistics.
5. National Center for Health Statistics (NCHS), "Health, U.S.," (Washington, D.C.: U.S. Government Printing Office, 1978).

Chapter 2

Historical Development of Health Care

T his chapter traces the historical development of health care for the aged and analyzes the process by which the elderly became a separate demographic group.

A considerable portion of the chapter is devoted to long-term care and the nursing home. Nursing home care consumes the largest amount of the health care dollar devoted to health care for the aged, this despite the fact that only about five percent of those 65 and over are residents of nursing homes.

The chapter also explores alternative forms of long-term care, such as home health care and day health care. These forms of health care can be either alternatives to nursing home care or supplemental services that help the elderly enhance the quality of their lives.

CONDITIONS PRIOR TO 1900

Historical analysis reveals that the concept of government financed long-term care evolved not necessarily and solely for the care of the aged, but rather for paupers who were unable to care for themselves. When the family could or would no longer care for the pauper, he or she became the government's responsibility by default and not necessarily by design. This responsibility ranged from providing financial assistance to families and individuals, to institutional relief programs such as almshouses, hospitals, workhouses, orphanages, and prisons. Families received government assistance for the care of a disabled or senile relative and even for the building of a separate cell or enclosure for a mentally ill person. This type of support system was developed during the colonial period and made no distinction between poverty due to physical disability and poverty resulting from economic distress.

In the seventeenth and eighteenth centuries, paupers were auctioned to persons willing to undertake their support at the lowest cost to the community. Among those auctioned were children, the disabled, the handicapped, the feebleminded, and the insane. Others were contracted to work in return for their care. It was not until after the American Revolution that the almshouse was considered the most suitable and least costly way to take care of the people in need. The 1843 Poor Law of England supported the concept of the almshouse as a means of assisting the poor. In Britain throughout the nineteenth century the view of long-term care institutions as a method of caring for the needy continued to gain acceptance despite the inhumane conditions maintained throughout these institutions. The British almshouse was described by Cohen:[1]

> The almshouse became the place of refuge for the impoverished, the insane, the feebleminded, the blind, the vagrant, and the sick, whether they were aged and abandoned, or so marginal as to be unable to make their way home. The almshouse pressed those who could work into servitude for it often had an associated workhouse. Poorhouses were operated cheaply on low appropriations, often no more than ten cents a day per resident, by persons who had to take out their own income from whatever they could save from the meager appropriations.

In the Colonies, when the formation of the states was barely underway, there were few voluntary organizations. The towns and counties gave financial support to such institutions.

Not until 1854 was there an indication that the government accepted responsibility to care for the disadvantaged and aged. In that year a bill for federal financing of the indigent insane was passed, signifying the first federal action dealing with public welfare. President Franklin Pierce vetoed the measure, maintaining that the federal government should not be involved in any welfare program.

With continued U.S. industrial development, a growing trend toward urbanization, and widespread unemployment, the almshouse continued to be the principal method of dealing with society's castoffs. Harshness in institutions continued and in fact was a matter of public policy, as noted in the New York State Department of Public Charities Report of 1875:[2]

> Care has been taken not to diminish the terrors of this last resort of poverty, "the almshouse," because it has been deemed better that a few should test the minimum rate at which existence can be preserved than that they would brave the shame of pauperism to gain admission to it.

By 1867 16 states had developed State Boards of Charities which began to inspect state welfare institutions and eventually assumed supervision of private institutions that received public funds. Ultimately, these State Boards of Charities developed standards of care for hospitals of the aged, for nursing homes, and for other welfare agencies.

IMPROVEMENTS IN THE TWENTIETH CENTURY

Social reform characterized the twenty-year period following the turn of the century. Public health dispensaries, hospitals for the well-to-do and for the indigent, and convalescent and rest homes were begun. A few states and cities attempted to improve the almshouse by developing systems of institutional classification, segregation of inmates and patients, and general program improvement.

As might be expected, welfare policy changed drastically with the Great Depression of the 1930s. Groups of Americans who once had frowned on public assistance now found themselves demanding it. In 1933 25 million people depended on relief for their sustenance. The growing need for assistance brought a turnabout in opinions concerning government involvement in public welfare programs. This shift in attitudes was soon reflected in policy outcomes.

The most important legislative action was the Social Security Act of 1935. Under this act, two systems were created: (1) a national retirement income system designed to provide income in lieu of wages to workers or their dependents when the worker retired or became disabled, and (2) a system of federal grants to assist the states in providing financial support to the aged, to dependent children, to the blind, and to the disabled. The early versions of the Social Security Act contained specific provisions against federal financial assistance to any kind of institutional setting. This prohibition reflected the distasteful perceptions of the traditional almshouse.

Before delving further into health care support systems, it is useful to examine how the elderly developed as a separate demographic segment of the overall population.

FORMATION OF THE ELDERLY AS A SEPARATE DEMOGRAPHIC GROUP

In 1975 well over 22 million people in the United States were over 65, a figure that approached 11 percent of the total population. Approximately equal to the entire population of Canada, this population group is larger than the entire population of the most heavily populated state.

This group has not always been so large. In 1900 the elderly amounted to 3.1 million, or about four percent of the population. By 2000 the group is expected to grow to about 30 million people, or about 12 percent of the population.

What sets this population group apart from the rest? There are three important factors: (1) political strength, (2) retirement, and (3) a relatively high need and consumption of health care services.

The political strength of the elderly is evidenced by the increasing amount of attention paid to them by politicians. The educated elderly have proven to be politically influential because they are able to organize themselves politically and get out the vote. As their numbers and their educational levels increase, their political power will also increase. Their governmental benefits are bound to increase, too, although there is a limit on the resources that society as a whole will be willing to spend on the elderly.

About 100 years ago Bismark selected 65 as the pension age for Germans. This decision is probably responsible for creating the elderly as a separate demographic group. In 1935 the United States Congress adopted 65 as the mandatory retirement age, making U.S. workers eligible for benefits under the new Social Security system. Since that time, American society and industry have had to accept 65 as the mandatory retirement age and have based many rules and plans around it.

In 1978 Congress extended a person's right to work to age 70. It was reasoned that the old mandatory retirement age had been set arbitrarily and although age 65 might once have been a reasonable age for retirement, it could no longer be justified, especially since the average person's life expectancy now extends a considerable period of time beyond it. Although we do not fully understand the aging process, it is known that people age at different rates and do not abruptly lose their ability or capability to work.

According to studies undertaken by federal agencies and academia, there is no indication that older workers are by definition poor workers. In fact, many studies reveal that older workers are superior in some instances. For a variety of reasons, older workers are usually more satisfied with their jobs than are younger workers, especially because older workers have more realistic goals and expectations than their younger colleagues. Furthermore, older workers will have settled into a more routine, stable lifestyle and are therefore likely to be steady, punctual employees with good attendance records.

Retirement syndrome, characterized by anxiety and depression, describes the physical and psychological consequences of mandatory retirement. Persons who develop this condition often complain of headaches and gastrointestinal problems, sleep more than they need to, and become irritable, nervous, and lethargic. Studies also indicate a correlation between mandatory retirement and the death rate. Early studies showed the mortality rate to be 30 percent higher than average for those who were forced into retirement at age 65. A forced change in lifestyle, caused by early retirement, can have a deleterious health effect, a theory considered by many, especially those in the field of gerontology, to be a legitimate concern.

Pension plans and insurance packages are currently geared to a retirement age of 65. However, those workers who can choose early retirement (such as firefighters, police officers, federal employees, etc.) quite often do so, collect their retirement checks, and in addition find new jobs that are less demanding.

Forced early retirement puts an economic burden on the American people. Those in the work force are particularly hard hit because that population segment is becoming proportionately smaller as compared to a growing retired population. The labor force must support those who are retired and, for the most part, nonproductive. The current pressure for earlier retirement is due to continuing high unemployment and comes primarily from younger workers and from employers who feel that rigid seniority and tenure rules give them very little flexibility. Contrary to popular belief, the pressure does not emanate from the older workers.

Extending the mandatory retirement age to 70 is a positive step, but 70 is merely another arbitrary figure. One compromise might be to allow the older worker to gradually withdraw from the labor force, probably at reduced levels of pay. This would encourage people to work as long as possible but not beyond their limits.

THE GROWTH OF PRIVATE NURSING HOME CARE

In the early twentieth century it was estimated that there were over 1,000 nursing homes in the United States. These homes were sponsored and supported largely by churches, fraternal organizations, social organizations, and philanthropic groups.

Applicants for admission had to comply with requirements in respect to physical condition, age, and property and residence mandates. In some instances membership in the sponsoring organization was also required. Some homes accepted only men, others only women, although many admitted both sexes. Nearly half made no financial demands, while others required weekly or monthly charges. Sometimes applicants had to pay an entrance fee ranging from about $500 to thousands of dollars. In some homes the residents were expected to "lend their services" for small duties around the home.

A clause in the Social Security Act set the groundwork for the present nursing home industry. As reported by Jacoby:[3]

> The little-noticed Social Security provision encouraged the conversion of private housing into profit making boarding homes for the elderly—the forerunner of today's nursing home industry. In the thirties, few planners foresaw the massive social needs that would arise when families began to slough off the responsibility for older relatives at the same time that medical advances were keeping unprece-

dented numbers of people alive into their 70s and 80s. And no one asked whether profit-making institutions were best designed to meet those needs.

Long-term institutional care changed little between the early 1900s and the 1930s. It has grown phenomenally since the 1930s. A 1939 Bureau of the Census study estimated that at that time there were twelve hundred facilities in the United States with twenty-five thousand beds. The 1954 inventory of all types of nursing homes and related facilities reported a total of three hundred thousand beds in eight thousand homes. The bulk of that growth reflected major postwar development of proprietary nursing homes to meet a significant backlogged demand. The demand continued unabated well into the late 1960s and early 1970s. Today there are approximately twenty-five thousand homes with a total capacity of over one million beds.

GOVERNMENT INVOLVEMENT IN CARE FOR THE AGED

Since World War II, a variety of explicit public policy enactments and events have been directed toward the issue of long-term care for the aged. A brief chronology of major executive and legislative decisions will show the extent and direction of national policy.[4]

1948   The Federal Security Agency (predecessor to the Department of Health, Education and Welfare) set up a task force on aging.

1950   Oscar Ewing, Director of the Federal Security Agency, called the first National Conference on Aging.

1953   Federal participation in the cost of assistance paid to indigent persons in private institutions was authorized. The prohibition against payment in public institutions continued.

States seeking federal participation in the cost of payments made to persons in private institutions were required to establish standards for such institutions.

1954   The Hill-Burton Program, for the first time, was given authority for aiding, through direct grants, public and other nonprofit sponsors in constructing and equipping nursing homes and related facilities.

1958   The Small Business Administration was authorized through the Small Business Act and the Small Business Investment Act to provide loans to nursing homes.

1959   The National Housing Act was amended to provide for mortgage insurance to private lenders to facilitate construction or rehabilitation of qualified proprietary nursing homes. (Subsequently this was extended to provide the same kinds of benefits to nonprofit facilities.)

1950s   Improvements in Social Security benefits were provided through significant increases and extensions of benefits to the disabled and through improvements in the earned income limitation provisions.

1960   Congress passes the Federal Assistance for the Aged Act to provide a program of federal financial assistance to the states to furnish care for the indigent and the medically indigent for a very wide variety of institutional and noninstitutional programs. Activities for the White House Conference on Aging were initiated and undertaken throughout the United States at local and state levels.

1961   White House Conference on Aging was held.

1965   Title 18 of the Social Security Act (Medicare) was passed, providing for, among other things, payment of posthospital care in extended care facilities.

Title 19, the Medical Assistance title, was passed, requiring states to include in their vendor payment programs inpatient and outpatient hospital services, laboratory and x-ray services, skilled nursing home care, and physician's services. Amendments to the Social Security Act were passed providing for grants to the states to aid in meeting the cost of care for persons 65 and over receiving the equivalent of skilled nursing care and active treatment in state hospitals for the mentally ill.

The Older Americans Act was passed, setting forth congressional policy concerning older Americans, defining the responsibilities of the state and federal governments, and providing for demonstration projects, research, and training programs.

1968   Congress authorized the President to call a White House Conference on Aging.

Intermediate care facilities were recognized as another type of facility that qualifies for federal participation in payments to indigent persons.

The Social Security Act was amended to strengthen the enforcement activities of the individual states in regard to nursing homes. The amendment provided that no federal matching funds be paid to any nursing home not fully meeting state requirements for licensure. In connection with the medical assistance program for skilled nursing home care, the act was amended to provide that states require a medical evaluation of each patient's needs prior to admission, followed by regular and periodic inspection (by an independent review team consisting of physicians and other health and social service personnel) of care being given to medical assistance patients in nursing homes.

1969   President Nixon called the White House Conference on Aging and initiated planning activities.

1971   The White House Conference on Aging was held. The Secretary of Health, Education and Welfare appointed a special assistant on nursing homes to deal with the problem.

The President made an address concerning nursing homes and federal actions designed to assist in correcting problems and abuses.

1972   Congress passed the Nutrition Bill for the elderly, authorizing an expenditure of $100 million to improve the nutrition of elderly Americans during fiscal 1973 and $150 million during fiscal 1974.

1973   Older Americans Act amendments:
- to provide $543.6 million for fiscal 1973-75
- to provide "such sums as necessary" for various federal programs
- shifted the Administration on Aging from HEW's Social and Rehabilitation section to the Office of HEW Secretary
- established National Clearinghouse for Information on Aging
- created Federal Council on Aging
- authorized grants for training and research in the field of aging
- authorized funds for the establishment of gerontology centers and for special transportation research projects.

Social Security Act amendments:
- extended Supplementary Security Income (SSI) coverage and increased benefits
- altered distribution of Social Security payments to increase old age and survivors payments and disability and hospital insurance
- extended Medicaid coverage to SSI recipients.

1974   Actions by Congress:
- increased nutrition funding

- authorized $35 million in grants to states for transportation programs for the elderly
- expanded the authority of the National Institute of Arthritis, Metabolism, and Digestive Diseases to "advance the attack on arthritis."

1975   Health Services Program begun:
- required that new and existing mental health centers seeking financial aid provide specialized services to the elderly
- authorized grants to establish, operate, or expand programs providing health care at home; priority areas were those with large numbers of elderly
- established national commissions to study mental health problems of the elderly.

Congress urged states and communities to provide health care services to the elderly at home to prevent undue institutionalization.

1976   Supplementary Security Income eligibility was broadened.

1977   Food Stamp program changed to allow some recipients to receive stamps without paying for them.

1978   Older Americans Act amendments:
- authorized funding for home-delivered meals programs
- expanded purpose of the act to include providing "a continuation of care" for the "vulnerable elderly."

THE NEXT STEP IN LONG-TERM CARE

Although demand for nursing home care is still quite extensive and many communities report virtually no vacancies, there are indications that nursing home bed growth will at least level out to a rate that reflects the growth of the elderly population. The reason for the reduced growth is the increasing demand for home and day health care. Although home and day care is not always a possibility for those elderly ill who require skilled nursing facility care, it is frequently adequate for many elderly now in health related facilities. The next few decades will see the development of programs that will offer combinations of nursing home care, home care, and day care for the elderly ill. Appropriate care will be determined by assessment and placement programs (see Chapter 8).

Home and day health care programs will have a much stronger likelihood of success if the elderly who can benefit from this type of care have a human support system of family, relatives, and friends on whom they can depend. There are indications that these human support systems will become more prevalent in the future. As Neugarten and Havighurst[5] point out, the last two decades have seen an increase in the percentage of older people who are married and living with spouses. In addition, the intergenerational family structure is expanding, with the four- and five-generation family becoming the norm. Furthermore, because of the 1950-60 baby boom, by the turn of the century the older person will have more surviving children on average than does the senior citizen living now.

All of the above changes, of course, assume that family members will be willing to provide emotional and physical support to their elderly parents and/or grandparents. A whole range of smaller studies point out that the family thus far has remained a strong and supportive institution for older people. It is safe to assume that this will hold true for the future.

Another factor that supports the growth of home and day health care is the development of senior citizen housing. The existence of high quality senior citizen housing provides the elderly with opportunities to socialize more easily and support each other, emotionally and physically. Providing home and day health care services to the elderly in a senior citizen housing project also provides considerable economies of scale by eliminating considerable travel and travel time for the health care providers.

CONCLUSIONS

It is apparent that since World War II our nation has shown increasing concern over the provision of adequate long-term care for the elderly. An historical acceptance of the nursing home as an acceptable method of providing care, plus a growing proportion of people over 65, have combined to make the proprietary nursing home the major dispensary of long-term care services. Spurred on by various legislative enactments (such as the Social Security Act), the nursing home industry has grown at a phenomenal pace. As a result, society is raising more and more questions about the cost and quality of services provided to the elderly and is looking more and more to alternative ways of caring for the elderly frail. These alternatives encompass various forms of home health care and day health care services.

NOTES

1. E. S. Cohen, "An Overview of Long-Term Care Facilities" in *A Social Work Guide for Long-Term Care Facilities,* edited by Elaine M. Brody, National Institute of Mental Health (Washington, D.C.: U.S. Government Printing Office, 1974), p. 13.

2. Ibid., p. 14.

3. Susan Jacoby, "Waiting for the End: On Nursing Homes," *The New York Times Magazine*, March 31, 1974.

4. E. S. Cohen, "An Overview of Long-Term Care Facilities" in *A Social Work Guide for Long-Term Care Facilities*, edited by Elaine M. Brody, National Institute of Mental Health (Washington, D.C.: U.S. Government Printing Office, 1974), p. 16-18.

5. B. L. Neugarten and R. J. Havighurst, "Aging and the Future," *Social Policy, Social Ethics, and the Aging Society* (Washington, D.C.: National Science Foundation, RANN-Research Applications Directorate, Division of Advanced Productivity, Research and Technology, 1976).

Chapter 3

The High Cost of Health Care

In the 1970s, the rapid increases in health care costs became a topic of major public concern. The rise in health care costs has been attributed not only to the health care industry, but also to the elderly. A close examination of how various facets of the health care system relate to rising health care costs will point out the impact of the older population on health care costs and the impact of rising health care costs on the elderly.

A PERIOD OF RISING EXPENDITURES

In the period between fiscal year 1966 and fiscal year 1977, total health care expenditures rose at a rate of 12 to 15 percent per year, reaching $162.6 billion or $767 per person in 1977, as shown in Table 3-1. Put yet another way, in 1977 health care expenditures amounted to 8.8 percent of the gross national product (GNP). Between 1976 and 1977 health care expenditures increased 12 percent, from $139.3 billion to $162.6 billion.

During the 1966–77 period, personal health care expenditures had been increasing 15 percent annually for persons age 65 and over as compared to 11 percent annually for those under 65. Therefore, in the ten-year period the proportion of health care expenditures for the aged had risen from 23 percent to 29 percent of total.[1]

In fiscal 1977, per capita health care spending for those 65 and over reached $1,745. The cost breaks down in this way: $769 spent for hospital care, $446 for institutional services, $302 for physicians' services, $121 for drugs and medical sundries, and $107 for miscellaneous services. This per capita figure was more than 2.5 times that for persons age 19 to 64 and nearly seven times that for persons under 19.

Although comprising only 11 percent of the population, the elderly accounted for 29 percent of personal health care spending, as shown in Table 3-2.

Table 3-1 National Health Expenditures Summary—1950–77

| Year | Total National Health Expenditures | | Per Capita National Health Expenditures |
	Dollars in Billions	Percent of GNP	
1950	$ 12.0	4.5	$ 78
1960	25.9	5.2	142
1970	69.2	7.2	334
1971	77.2	7.6	368
1972	86.7	7.8	410
1973	95.4	7.7	447
1974	106.3	7.8	495
1975	122.2	8.4	564
1976	139.3	8.6	638
1977	162.6	8.8	767

Source: National Center for Health Statistics, *Health, U.S.* (Washington, D.C.: U.S. Government Printing Office, 1978).

Table 3-2 Personal Health Care Expenditures by Source of Funds and Age Group—Fiscal Year 1977

| Source of Funds | Age Group | | | Total |
	Under 19	19–64	65 and over	
Federal	$ 3.22B (18%)	$13.34B (16%)	$23.54B (57%)	$ 40.10B (28%)
State and Local	$ 2.33B (13%)	$10.84B (13%)	$ 4.13B (10%)	$ 17.30B (12%)
Private	$12.35B (69%)	$59.22B (71%)	$13.63B (33%)	$ 85.20B (60%)
Total	$17.9B (13%)	$83.4B (58%)	$41.3B (29%)	$142.6B (100%)

Note: Percentage figures are by age group categories.
Source: Social Security Bulletin 42-1 (Washington, D.C.: U.S. Government Printing Office, 1979).

Table 3-3 Per Capita Health Care Expenditures for the Aged—Fiscal
Year 1977

Sources of Funds	Types of Care			Total
	Hospital	Physician	Other	
Medicare	$572	$168	$ 22	$ 762
	(74%)	(56%)	(3%)	(44%)
Medicaid	$ 27	$ 9	$255	$ 291
	(4%)	(3%)	(38%)	(17%)
Other Public Programs	$ 79	$ 3	$ 33	$ 115
	(10%)	(1%)	(5%)	(6%)
Private Sources	$ 91	$122	$364	$ 577
	(12%)	(40%)	(54%)	(33%)
Totals	$769	$302	$674	$1745
	(44%)	(17%)	(39%)	(100%)

Note: Percentage increases are by types of care.
Source: Social Security Bulletin 42-1 (Washington, D.C.: U.S. Government Printing Office, 1979).

In contrast, health care expenditures for those under age 19 had dropped from 15 percent of the total in 1970 to less than 13 percent in 1977.[2]

A large portion of medical care costs for the elderly is paid for by public funds, as shown on Table 3-3. One source of public money is Medicare, established in 1966 to give the elderly some relief from the financial burden of high medical bills. In fiscal 1977 the Medicare program paid 44 percent of these medical bills, or $18 billion.

PUBLIC HEALTH EXPENDITURE SUPPORT

The Medicare program was not created to provide total coverage for all medical care costs for the aged. Actually Medicare is very similar to private health insurance, with emphasis on coverage of hospital care and physicians' services. Seventy-four percent of hospital care expense and 56 percent of the cost of physicians' services are covered by Medicare. However, nursing home care is covered only if it is required after a hospital stay. In 1977 Medicare provided only about three percent of nursing home care expenditures.[3] As with most private health insurance coverage, routine physical examinations, dental care, and vision care are excluded.

In 1977 Medicaid helped 3.6 million low-income elderly, providing them with $6.9 billion of health care. This figure equaled 17 percent of all health care costs for the elderly.

In addition to Medicare and Medicaid, several other public sources of funds are available. The Veterans Administration provides health care for eligible veterans and their dependents, while the Department of Defense provides health care to retired military persons and dependents. The federal government spent $1.1 billion for these two programs. Mental hospital care for some of the aged is financed by state funds. Together, the various government sources supplied about eight percent of these expenses.

When all the government programs' expenditures are added, they amount to about 67 percent of the medical costs paid for the elderly. Private health insurance provides less than six percentage points of the remaining 33 percent. The balance of 27 percent, or $463 per person, is paid from an individual's own income or family aid.[4]

It is interesting to note that before 1966, only 25 percent of total health care expenditures were paid for by government funds. Since that time government expenditures have risen almost 18 percent annually, and private spending has risen by about 10 percent annually.[5] During the same period per capita expenditures for the aged increased 13 percent annually, while direct or "out-of-pocket" payments by the elderly increased six percent annually. If insurance premiums paid by the elderly are included in the "out-of-pocket" expenses, the figure is 6.6 percent annual rate. In the same period, per capita income for the aged went up ten percent a year. Therefore, "out-of-pocket" expenses as a percentage of average income declined from 15 to 11 percent.[6]

There are essentially two reasons why the government has had to assume an ever-increasing share of health care expenses for the aged: (1) decline of family support and (2) increases in numbers.

FAMILY AND HOUSEHOLD STATUS OF THE ELDERLY

The decline in family support has to date been moderate. Most persons age 65 and over still live in families. Although the proportion of older men and women living in families differs greatly, the number of older men and women living in families is about the same, 7.6 million men versus 7.5 million women. In 1978 a full 82 percent of all elderly men lived in families and 77 percent maintained their own families. Among elderly women, however, only 57 percent still lived in families and only 36 percent still had spouses (see Figure 3–1).

In addition, a large proportion of older persons maintain their own households either alone or with nonrelatives. Most older women who live alone are widows. Figures in 1978 show that 52 percent of women 65 years and over and

Figure 3-1 Percent of Persons 65 Years and Over, by Marital Status and Sex—March 1978

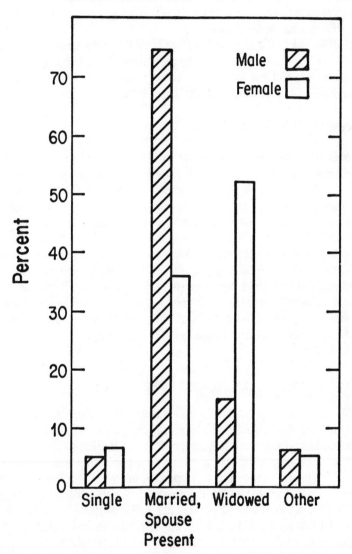

Source: Bureau of the Census, "Social and Economic Characteristics of the Older Population, 1978" (Washington, D.C.: U.S. Government Printing Office, 1979).

69 percent of those 75 years and over were widowed. Among men, the corresponding proportions were 14 percent and 23 percent, respectively. Note also that women not only outnumber men among the older population in general but also among the institutionalized elderly.

In recent years the husband-wife dyad has been declining because of higher divorce rates. If this trend continues, the proportion of elderly living without traditional family support will increase even more sharply than expected, necessitating broader public financing of health care costs.

INCREASING NUMBER OF ELDERLY WOMEN

The number of women 65 and over has increased faster than the number of men in the same age group. Specifically, since 1970 the annual increase for women amounts to 22 percent, as compared to ten percent for men. Interestingly, the number of elderly men and women were about equal at the beginning of this century. At present, elderly women outnumber elderly men by 4.5 million—14.3 million women and 9.8 million men.[7]

At age 65 life expectancy is about 14 years for men but 18 years for women. As a result, there were 146 elderly women per 100 elderly men in 1977, and the gap continues to grow with age. Put another way, of the 1.2 million older people who died in 1976 at a rate of 54 per 1,000, 67 were men and 46 were women.[8] Assuming that the mortality trends do not change in the future, 82 percent of female babies will live to the age of 65, as compared to only 68 percent of male babies.

CAUSES OF RISING HEALTH CARE EXPENDITURES

Since 1900 the elderly population increased nearly 700 percent (an eight-fold increase), while the total population increased about 200 percent. Since 1970 the number of elderly increased 20 percent, from 20 million to about 24 million. In 1900 the proportion of elderly to the total population was 4.1 percent (see Table 3-4). The proportion rose to 11 percent in 1978. The declining death rate has been another factor. In 1965 the death rate for the elderly was 60 persons per 1,000, as compared to 54 persons per 1,000 in 1975.

It is projected that by 2020 the elderly may comprise as much as 20 percent of total population. At that point the median age of the population will be 37, as compared to 29 in 1980. Not only is the total number of persons age 65 and over increasing; the number of very old is increasing even more rapidly. For example, from 1950 to 1975 the total U.S. population rose by less than 50 percent. However, the number of persons age 75 to 84 doubled, and the number of those 85 years and over more than tripled. The projection is that the number of those 85 and over will increase by an additional 80 percent by the year 2000.

Table 3-4 Older Population Statistics During the Twentieth Century

Year	Number (in Millions)	Percent of Total	Men (in Millions)	Women (in Millions)	Number of Women to 100 Men
1900	3.1M	4.1%	1.6M	1.5M	98
1930	6.6M	5.4%	3.3M	3.3M	100
1970	20.0M	9.8%	8.4M	11.6M	139
1977	23.5M	10.9%	9.6M	13.9M	146
2000	31.8M	12.5%	12.7M	19.1M	150

Source: U.S. Bureau of the Census, "Social and Economic Characteristics of the Older Population, 1978 " (Washington, D.C.: U.S. Government Printing Office, 1979).

Average life expectancy has also increased. In 1900 average life expectancy for Americans at birth was 47.3 years. In 1976 it was 73 years. The average white man at age 65 can expect to live nearly 13.8 additional years, and the average white woman can expect 18.1 additional years, as shown in Table 3-5. Most of this increase is due to the decline in infant mortality and the improvement in elderly mortality. Another factor, not as significant, is immigration.

Because older persons tend to suffer from chronic conditions, many elderly are limited in their activities or are hospitalized more frequently and for longer periods. People age 65 to 69 require about 3,000 days of short-stay hospital care per year per 1,000 persons. People in their late 70s require 4,700 days per 1,000 persons, while those over 85 require, 8,300 days per 1,000 persons.[9]

Table 3-5 Expected Number of Years Remaining at Age 65 by Race, and Sex—Selected Years, 1900–76

	White		Negro and Other	
Year	Male	Female	Male	Female
1901	11.5	12.2	10.4	11.4
1950	12.8	15.0	12.8	14.5
1974	13.4	17.6	13.4	16.7
1975	13.7	18.1	13.7	17.5
1976	13.7	18.1	13.8	17.6

Sources: National Center for Health Statistics, *Health, U.S.* (Washington, D.C.: U.S. Government Printing Office, 1978).
Bureau of the Census, *Statistical Abstracts of U.S.* (Washington, D.C.: U.S. Government Printing Office, 1978).

In the period between 1960 and 1970, the proportion of elderly living in institutions increased 25 percent, from four percent (1960) to five percent (1970). However, use of nursing home services increases with age. The elderly require about 16,000 days of nursing home care per year per 1,000 persons; those age 85 and over require 86,400 days per 1,000 persons per year.[10] The surgical rate for the aged increased 44 percent between 1965–66 and 1975–76. Physician visits are also higher for the elderly than for the younger population, mainly because of the chronic nature of conditions. During 1975–76, youths under 18 years of age averaged 4.1 visits per person annually, as compared to 6.7 visits for the elderly.[11]

However, there was no significant rise in the rate of physician visits for the elderly between 1965–75, averaging 6.6 visits per year. A reason for this constancy is that the decrease in physician visits by nonpoor elderly cancelled the increase in visits by poor elderly. Indeed, between 1968–74, the hospital admission rate increased, but with a decline in the length of stay.[12] Even before 1966, the elderly accounted for nearly 2.5 times as many days in short-time hospital visits and a third more physician visits.

Many people believe that the tremendous rise in health care expenditures, especially government's share, is due purely to the increased use of medical care by the aged. This is true to some extent. But there are other factors involved. First of all, medical science and technology has advanced a great deal, enabling the elderly to take advantage of more complex and more expensive procedures and medications. Furthermore, medical care has grown more intensified, with physicians using every possible means to treat patients, even the dying. Finally, there are simply not many inexpensive long-term care facilities.

EFFECTS OF PRICE CHANGES ON HEALTH CARE EXPENDITURES

Inflation has been the major factor responsible for the increase in health care expenditures between 1950–75, as shown in Table 3-6. During that period, total expenditures rose at an average annual rate of 10.4 percent. A still larger increase occurred between 1974 and 1977. After adjusting for inflation, the increase averaged 9 percent per year, accounting for nearly half of the total increase.[13] In that three-year period (1974–77), price changes accounted for 80 percent of total change. This was a result of President Nixon's Economic Stabilization Program (see Table 3-6).[14]

The annual growth rate has not been uniform among the various components of national health care expenditures. Hospital costs rose at an annual rate of 11 percent. Even more discouraging, in recent years hospital room rates have been increasing at twice the rate of nonmedical items. For instance, in 1976 the hos-

Table 3-6 Percentage Increases in Personal Health Care Expenditures—Selected Periods, 1950–76

	Causes of Increases			
Fiscal Year Period	Changes in Prices	Changes in Composition of Services	Changes in Population	Total
1950–65	43.8%	35.2%	21.0%	100%
1965–71	49.9%	41.2%	8.9%	100%
1971–74	43.1%	49.0%	7.9%	100%
1974–76	78.3%	15.9%	5.7%	100%

Source: Anne R. Somers, "The High Cost of Health Care for the Elderly: Diagnosis, Prognosis, and Some Suggestions for Therapy," *Journal of Health Politics, Policy and Law* (Summer 1978): 163-180.

pital room rate rose by 16.1 percent, as compared with an increase of 7.8 percent for all nonmedical items.[15] This phenomenal increase in room rates slowed to 13 percent by the beginning of 1977, remaining constant since then. During the 12 months ending March 1979, $78.3 billion was spent on hospital care, a 12.2 percent increase. In calendar year 1978, the increase was 12 percent. By March 1979, $13.6 billion had been spent for physicians' services, up 13.9 percent. Nursing home care expenditures had increased by 17.3 percent, reaching $16.3 billion. Other types of personal health care spending—such as for dental treatment, drugs, and eyeglasses—also showed increases.[16]

CONCLUSIONS

There is little doubt that rising health care costs will remain an important area of concern for legislators, administrators, and policy makers. Since the elderly as a group are the highest per capita health care consumers, it is also clear that their health care consumption will continue to be analyzed and evaluated.

Unfortunately, it is unlikely that health care consumption can be reduced. If anything, total health care expenditures for the elderly will undoubtedly increase, because the number of elderly in the total population is growing. In addition, as the many unmet health care needs of the elderly are underwritten by future public financing, this will further increase the per capita health care costs of this group.

Barring some major scientific breakthrough that results in reduced health care needs and increased health, there is only one way direction for health care expenditures to go in the next several years—up.

NOTES

1. R. M. Gibson and C. R. Fisher, "Age Difference in Health Care Spending Fiscal Year 1977," *Social Security Bulletin* 42-1 (Washington, D.C.: U.S. Government Printing Office, January 1979), p. 3-16.

2. Ibid.

3. Ibid.

4. Ibid.

5. National Center for Health Statistics, *Health, U.S.* (Washington, D.C.: U.S. Government Printing Office, 1978).

6. Gibson and Fisher, "Age Difference in Health Care Spending," p. 3-16.

7. Bureau of the Census, "Social and Economic Characteristics of the Older Population, 1978" (Washington, D.C.: U.S. Government Printing Office, 1979).

8. Administration on Aging, "Facts about Older Americans, 1978" (Washington, D.C.: U.S. Government Printing Office, 1979).

9. Gibson and Fisher, "Age Difference in Health Care Spending," p. 3-16.

10. Ibid.

11. National Center for Health Statistics, *Health, U.S.*

12. Marion Gornick, "Ten Years of Medicare: Impact on the Covered Population," *Social Security Bulletin* 39 (July 1976): 3-21.

13. National Center for Health Statistics, *Health, U.S.*

14. A. R. Somers, "The High Cost of Health Care for the Elderly: Diagnosis, Prognosis, and Some Suggestions for Therapy," *Journal of Health Politics, Policy and Law* (Summer, 1978): 163-180.

15. D. R. Waldo, "Health Care Financing Trends," Health Care Financing Administration (Washington, D.C.: U.S. Government Printing Office, 1979).

16. Ibid.

Chapter 4

Information, Referral, and Support Services for the Elderly

Local government, especially in the more urban areas, is becoming increasingly aware of its responsibilities to provide or arrange for a variety of support services tailored to the needs of the elderly. Recognition of this responsibility has usually resulted in the creation of an office or department in the local government devoted to and responsible for the needs of the elderly. Usually these divisions are known as Offices for the Aging, Departments of Senior Services, and so on.

There are many factors to be evaluated in determining what services are needed by older people. It has been estimated that about one-quarter of the elderly live alone, that about one-quarter have incomes at or below the poverty level, and that well over one-third have one or more activity-limiting conditions. Frequently these three segments overlap, and it is this resulting group that particularly needs assistance.

Although many elderly with activity-limiting conditions are able to sustain a minimum daily living standard, there are many others who require assistance in one or more areas, such as meal preparation, housekeeping, and shopping. Others require assistance with transportation, medical treatment, social activities, and so forth. Still others are completely homebound and need home health care services. This chapter reviews the various services available to the elderly.

COMMUNITY ORGANIZATIONS

Community support services are designed to help older persons remain in their customary environments, usually their own homes and neighborhoods. The overall goal is to minimize their chances of relocation and to defer various levels of dependency, especially institutionalization, for as long as possible.

Community support services includes all those services that may be required to complement the comprehensiveness of the overall system of health-social services. For example, it promotes the use of existing programs and provides opportunities for the elderly to enhance the quality of their lives. It serves to generate activity programs and coordinates services offered by various government, charitable, and profit-motivated organizations. It informs individuals about appropriate types of assistance and makes referrals as needed. In addition, it may try to identify hard-to-reach persons and help them gain access to needed services. Transportation facilitation is also part of many modern support efforts.

The senior citizen center provides a setting for organized activities and recreation and serves as a meeting place for the elderly. It usually offers a gamut of services such as nutritional programs and shuttle services, makes arrangements for medical examinations, and provides counseling regarding personal and legal problems, the aging process, and civil rights. To augment its programs, the senior citizen center establishes certain working relationships with other agencies.

The multipurpose center is an extension of the senior citizen center concept. The multipurpose center offers a complete range of services at a central location and provides limited services at surrounding satellite centers. Although the idea was designed to apply to the elderly, there is potential application for all age groups in the community.

A strategically placed multipurpose center can reduce fragmentation of services. However, the multipurpose concept is difficult to implement because of the variety of organizations currently providing their own services. Most of these organizations are reluctant to yield control. Communities must organize the multitude of organizations in a manner consistent with the operational requirements of the multipurpose center and with the needs of the people it serves.

COMPONENTS OF HEALTH AND SOCIAL SERVICES

The broad range of health and social services can be grouped into maintenance services, personal care services, supportive medical services, medical services, and personal planning. Financial support for these services will be discussed later in this book.

It is useful to outline in detail the various components of health and social services. This outline is based on Brody's organization of those services.[1]

   A.   *Maintenance Service*
       1.   *Income maintenance* is available through public assistance, social security, veterans benefits, unemployment compensation, workmen's compensation, and food stamps.

2. *Personal maintenance*
   a) Public assistance is available under Titles 1 or 16 of the Social Security Act (Old Age Assistance). States are authorized to provide homemaker services as part of social services to the aged.
   b) Older Americans Act provides assistance under Title 3 of the Older Americans Act. Grants are made to homemaker and nutrition programs, including Meals on Wheels.
   c) Veterans Administration provides special support to handicapped veterans and their dependent survivors. This support can be used to purchase homemaker services.

B. *Personal Care*
   1. *Medicare* includes personal care as a reimbursable item only when furnished through a home-health agency primarily engaged in delivering skilled nursing care, on a part-time intermittent basis. Reimbursement is provided only if it can be demonstrated that personal care is needed and that the patient is severely limited in function. The physician must regularly certify that the patient is sick enough to need the service and that the patient's condition demands only part-time intermittent care.
   2. *Medicaid* in several states provides reimbursement for medical assistance programs such as personal health care services.
   3. *Public assistance* in some states provides personal care services through a "special need" grant as an addition to the income maintenance grant.
   4. *Local public health* services may include personal care as part of their home-health program. Hospital-based home-health programs and neighborhood health centers may also offer personal care services, although they usually depend on Medicare or Medicaid for reimbursement. Private health insurance policies rarely cover such services.

C. *Supportive Medical Services*
   Supportive medical services are those aspects of home-health care such as nursing, physical therapy, occupational therapy, or speech therapy.
   1. *Medicare* provides reimbursement under the same conditions as described in this outline under B1 (Personal Care).
   2. *Medicaid* in some states reimburses coordinated home care programs, particularly when they are extensions of hospital service.
   3. *State rehabilitation agencies* may provide vendor payments for these services if they are part of a plan to make the client self-sufficient. This is a state-federal matching funds program.

D. *Medical Services*

Medical services for the aged are financed largely under Title 18 (Medicare) and Title 19 (Medicaid) of the Social Security Act. Medicaid is commonly only available for very low income groups.

1. *Hospital insurance (Medicare)* is provided through Part A of Title 18. It provides protection for covered services to any person 65 or over who is entitled to social security or railroad retirement benefits. Hospital insurance benefits are paid to participating hospitals, to extended care facilities (skilled nursing homes), and to related providers of health care to cover the reasonable cost of medically necessary services furnished to individuals entitled under this program.

    The hospital insurance program pays a large part of the cost of up to 90 days care during each benefit period. Each benefit period begins with the first day of hospitalization and ends 60 days after discharge from a hospital or extended care facility (ECF). Hospital insurance also pays part of the cost of care for up to 100 days (during the benefit period) in a participating ECF when admission follows a hospital stay of at least 3 days. In addition, the program covers up to 100 home health visits in the 12-month period following discharge from a hospital or ECF.

2. *Supplementary medical insurance (SMI)* is a voluntary medical insurance program financed by monthly premiums from enrollees and a matching payment from federal general revenues. It provides payment for 80 percent of the reasonable charges for physician's services, outpatient hospital services, medical supplies and services, home health services, outpatient physical therapy, and other health care services. It includes 100 home health visits each year, diagnostic tests, x-rays, radium and radioactive isotope therapy, ambulance services, prosthetic devices, and rental of durable medical equipment.

    An annual $60 deductible must be met before benefits begin. Thereafter, Medicare pays 80 percent of the charge for covered services. The beneficiary is responsible for the $60 deductible and for 20 percent of the cost of covered services.

    Application for the program is made through the local social security office within three months after the 65th birthday, or within three years of the first opportunity to sign up for medical insurance.

3. *Medicaid* coverage varies by state both as to eligibility and extent of benefits. Those aged receiving or eligible for categorical assistance are eligible for the medical program provided under

Title 19. The elderly with marginal incomes above the public assistance eligibility limits are often provided with the same amount or with a reduced amount of benefits. The usual arrangement for the medically and categorically needy is for the state to buy in on their behalf for Part B of Title 18, and to supplementally fund the co-pay aspects of Parts A and B.

4. *Blue Cross and private insurance* offer policies that cover the contributory aspect of the 20 percent of the cost required. Often private insurance companies provide similar types of coverage.

E. *Personal Planning*

The counseling offered by social workers, family agencies, mental health centers, home-health care agencies, vocational rehabilitation agencies, and protective services for adults unable (or unwilling) to manage their own affairs falls under the auspices of a multitude of government and charitable programs. The range and quality of these services varies widely and represents what is available in the community.

Information, referral, transportation, and outreach services are similarly diverse. Usually funding is available under service granting mechanisms such as Office of Economic Opportunity (OEO), Health, Education and Welfare (HEW), or Older Americans Act (OAA), and under service sections of Titles 1, 16, and 19 of the Social Security Act.

The next section illustrates the most logical way to organize, coordinate, and/or supply the services outlined above.

A TYPICAL LOCAL GOVERNMENT OFFICE FOR THE AGING

This section describes the programs and services typically provided by an Office of the Aging in a large urban area in the Northeastern United States.

The Office for the Aging performs an important function in transmitting information and referring clients to its own programs as well as to those offered by other agencies. Major agencies to which clients are referred include the County Department of Social Services, Legal Aid Bureau, Legal Counseling for the Elderly, Planning and Community Services, United Way, In-Home Support Services Corporation, Meals on Wheels, Catholic Charities, and others. The services range from counseling to home-delivered meals.

The primary targets of the Office for the Aging are those persons over 60 years of age who are isolated, have a low income level, or have physical or mental functional impairments and are considered to be at high risk to institutionalization.

The Office for the Aging offers many programs and services to the older segment of the population. These programs and services include:

- Transportation—maintains and updates a system of escort service for older persons.

- Information and referral—provides current information on services available to older persons.

- Multiservice senior centers—provides aid to senior citizen centers, including help in offering a broader range of services.

- Nutritional services—provides a balanced home-delivered meal to those elderly unable to cook for themselves.

- In-home services—provides homemaker and home health aide services to those ineligible under Medicaid, Title 20, or private services.

- Legal services—provides legal counseling services.

- Personal contact—provides personal contact, escort, and chore services to alleviate loneliness and isolation.

- Complimentary card—assists the elderly by stretching the purchasing power of their limited income.

- Outreach—seeks out and identifies hard-to-reach individuals so that they can gain access to services.

- Protective services—assists elderly persons who are unable to protect their own interests or meet their own needs and who have no one willing or able to help.

- Safety—helps protect the elderly from crime.

- Institutionally related services—provides Day Care and Respite as two institutionally-related services.

- Employment—develops jobs and provides employment opportunities.

- R.S.V.P.—provides administrative support to Retired Senior Volunteer Program.

- Education—increases community awareness through educational services.

- Recreation—provides opportunities for recreational activities.

- Housing improvement program—contracts with Catholic Charities to operate Housing Improvement Services.

Each program and service listed above is designed to meet the needs of particular subclasses in the elderly populations. The programs are implemented in compliance with all applicable federal, state, and local laws.

EFFECTIVENESS OF INFORMATION AND REFERRAL SERVICES

An extensive HEW-supported demonstration project to offer information and referral services took place in the state of Wisconsin during the mid-1970s. The study involved the demonstration project and a subsequent evaluation of the effectiveness of the services provided. The results of this study were reported by Long[2] for the period beginning October 1, 1973 and ending September 30, 1974.

The researchers considered that basically two services—information giving and referral—were provided as part of the demonstration aspects of the study. Information giving was defined as providing information about services and programs. It included some effort to obtain background materials about the potential client in order to determine his or her eligibility for the services of a specific provider. Referral was defined as making an appointment with the appropriate service provider by the Information and Referral Center on behalf of the caller.

The demonstration project provided information and referral services by telephone through a dozen Information and Referral Centers. The activities of the centers were largely information giving. Although referral services (including the making of an appointment) were offered, less than one percent of the callers accepted referral appointments. Of those who did accept the referral appointment, 82 percent contacted the recommended facility. Approximately 71 percent of those receiving information contacted the recommended facility. Callers who accepted referral appointments required about ten minutes more staff time than those who only were given information. About 61 percent of all calls were handled within ten minutes, with 60 percent being completed during the initial contact. Over 87 percent of all callers were helped within one day of their contact with an Information and Referral Center.

Once the centers had become known in the communities and the center staffs had been trained, the overall cost for providing basic information and referral services amounted to less than five dollars per call (in 1973–74 dollars). Almost 90 percent of those who contacted a program or service recommended by the centers indicated that they felt they had been sent to the right place. Approximately 17 percent of those who contacted a recommended service or program were sent elsewhere for help with their problems.

These statistics clearly indicate the value and need of the services that can be provided to the elderly by an Information and Referral Service.

CONCLUSIONS

It is now widely accepted that society has an obligation to help support the elderly. Assistance is best offered as a preventive service that provides information, referral, and support. Isolation of elderly persons as a result of retirement and lack of regular social contact often leads to declining health. This declining health can lead to other problems. It is in those cases where information, referral, and support services become increasingly important to the elderly.

Support programs such as those provided by community and senior citizen centers provide the elderly with a source for information and a local site for social gatherings. Federal, state, and local government-supported agencies complement these centers by facilitating programs designed to enable older persons to achieve or maintain independence and self-sufficiency.

NOTES

1. S. J. Brody, "Long–Term Care in the Community," in *A Social Work Guide for Long–Term Care Facilities,* edited by Elaine M. Brody, National Institutes of Mental Health (Washington, D.C.: U.S. Government Printing Office, 1974), p. 46-62.

2. Nicholas Long, *Information and Referral Services: Research Findings,* Vol. 1. DHEW Publication No. (OHDS) 77-16251, Office of Human Development, Administration on Aging, 1977.

Chapter 5

Institutional vs. Noninstitutional Care for the Elderly*

Abstract. The question of institutionalization vs. home care of the aged in need of medical care has been debated extensively. The arguments for deinstitutionalization have stressed the issue of cost. Home care is felt to be more cost efficient than institutional care. In this paper, both sides of the issue are investigated in detail by drawing on published conference proceedings and empirical studies reported in the literature.

Discussions concerning health care for the elderly usually begin with the subject of quality of care and end with the bleak topic of costs. This is precisely what happened during a 1976 series of regional public hearings on home health care sponsored by the Department of Health, Education and Welfare.[1]

While there were a number of concerns expressed by the witnesses, the major thrust of the testimony indicated a need for an expanded and coordinated range of high quality home care services as part of an essential continuum of health, social and support services. There was a consensus on the need for broader coverage of homemaker and home health aide services by all third-party payment programs. Another area of concern was for transportation services, home-delivered meals and nutrition services, and some mechanism for coordinating the delivery of round-the-clock services at the local level.

Since many persons offering testimony were from professions associated with medical care for the elderly, there was a high degree of concern expressed

Source: C. Carl Pegels, *Journal of Health Politics, Policy and Law*, Vol. 2, Summer 1980. Copyright 1980 by the Department of Health Administration, Duke University, pp. 205-212.

*This chapter was written with the assistance of research assistants Steven Gabor, Paul J. Gworek, Peter Markulis, and Kyle McNeil.

about patients' needs which witnesses felt should determine eligibility for services. Many witnesses argued for the elimination of artificial barriers to obtaining needed home health services: In the three day prior hospitalization requirement, homebound requirements, and restrictions that care be intermittent and restorative.

COST CONTAINMENT VS. EXPANDED SERVICES

What is most intriguing about the regional hearings is the fact that although most participants argued for increased services, they agreed that cost containment was imperative in health care delivery. Home health care was perceived by the majority of witnesses not only as socially beneficial in fostering independence but as less costly than institutionalized care. They also believed that a certain percentage (25 to 40 percent) of persons are institutionalized because of the lack of alternative home health care and community support services.

What must be considered, however, is that expansion of home health care may not decrease the institutionalized population of elderly persons but simply add a new layer, the home bound elderly, to the public health delivery system. Hence, cost containment cannot be the only criterion used in fostering home care and some home health advocates, such as the Columbia Conference on Home-Health Services,[2] stress the desirability of home health with regard to the importance of family, physical-emotional and mental health, and freedom of choice. However, the widening acceptance of institutionalization of elderly persons has occurred because of changes in cultural moves and, more immediately, because of governmental support through Medicaid and Medicare. Willingly or not, the family has abdicated its responsibility toward parents. It is now socially acceptable for parents to enter nursing homes or similar institutions, either of their own accord, or by being "placed" there by the children.

With regard to government financing, a recent report published by the Congressional Budget Office[3] noted that as the main source of funding for long-term care, Medicaid spending for nursing homes totalled $5.6 billion in 1977. Care in skilled nursing facilities is a mandated basic Medicaid service for all eligible individuals over 21 years of age. In nineteen states, nursing homes account for the bulk of Medicaid expenditures. And Medicaid is by no means the only source of public funding for long-term health care for the elderly; Medicare, Veteran's benefits, Supplemental Security Income, Social Services and various state and local programs also contribute considerable sums.

NONINSTITUTIONAL CARE—A DESIRED OPTION

As the regional surveys report, noninstitutional care for many elderly people is the desired option in terms of social, emotional and mental well-being.[4] Acknowledging the fact that most elderly persons would prefer to live outside the institutional setting and that it may, indeed, be cost-effective to do so in terms of public spending, one still must ask: Where will the discharged elderly go? A second question, contingent upon the first is: Who will pay?

Critics of the present system concur that the single largest factor behind the lack of adequate or appropriate long-term care for a large number of elderly is the general lack of formal alternatives to institutional care. Once it is determined that a person is incapable of living at home without some form of additional support or health care, the question of whether he or she will remain in the community depends upon the existence of social support (generally family or close friends), the adequacy of financial resources and the availability of noninstitutional health and social services. Unfortunately, many of the elderly are poor and either have no spouse or child(ren) to assist them. Furthermore, families may merely refuse or be unable to assist the elderly person due to distance, living facilities, family structure, and financial limitations. In any event, if there is no social support available from family or friends, the grim alternative is a nursing home, in which long-term care services are heavily subsidized by the government.

While the public may well have to pay the bill for a complete range of noninstitutionalized services for the elderly person such as nutritional, recreational, medical, transportation, and housing services, a cogent argument based on equity and dignity can still be made for providing them. In terms of equity, it would seem that persons inappropriately[5] placed in nursing facilities are creating an excessive cost burden on the public, thus drawing support away from such care even when it is appropriate. Also, inappropriate institutionalization encourages more of the same, driving a bitter wedge between those families willing to assist in supporting an elderly person and those unwilling to do so.

Regarding dignity, as stated above, institutionalization usurps the older person of his or her sense of worth and independence.

The establishment of mechanisms to curb inappropriate placement in institutionalized facilities confronts a dilemma: the proportion of elderly population itself is growing and the upper half of the elderly population (75 and over)—those who are most likely to have chronic conditions—are the fastest growing segment. This growing population will not only put increasing pressure on institutionalized facilities, but also on alternate forms of care, principally home care. Hence, the potential demand for long-term care is estimated to increase from 5.5 to 9.9 million presently, to 6.3 to 11.1 million in 1980, and 7.4 to 12.5 million in 1985. Furthermore, it is estimated[6] that many of the five to ten million adults who might have needed some form of long-term care in 1975 were not receiving it. As the Kahanas[7] point out, the central problem in geriatrics today is the development of services assisting a growing number of noninstitutionalized, impeded elderly.

COST SAVINGS FROM DE-INSTITUTIONALIZATION

Having discussed qualitative aspects of institutionalization v. alternative services, this section concentrates on costs. In its 1977 *Annual Report*[8] the Minneapolis Age and Opportunity Center (MAO) of the National Institute on Aging presented results of case studies of the comparative costs of institutional and in-home care. Three of these studies are presented to illustrate the potential monetary benefits to be derived from the utilization of in-home services. Supportive evidence from other countries also will be reviewed briefly.

Case A

Mrs. O. is a 77 year old who was hospitalized when an infected toe had to be amputated. Mrs. O. wanted to return home as soon as possible, so a MAO counselor, in consultation with her doctor, arranged supportive services—home delivered meals, homemaking services, nursing, an outpatient medical follow-up, transportation, and counseling—that enabled her to leave the hospital earlier than would have been possible because of the foot care she needed.

Cost if the Client had been Hospitalized 4 Extra Days

Average Basic Cost of Hospitalization per day at $175/day for 4 days	$700
Less Cost of MAO Services	−71
Savings to Government	$629

Case B

Mr. A., who became a double amputee as a result of a car accident, could not adjust to institutionalization beyond the time necessary to recover. As a proud individualist, he emphatically stated that he would not allow a deteriorating body to limit the scope of his intellectual or emotional life. A MAO counselor assessed the problems with Mr. A. to set up on-going services and provide relief of the most pressing ones immediately.

Costs if the Client had been Institutionalized
from June 20, 1974-Dec. 31, 1977

Average Basic Cost of Nursing Home Care at $725/mon. for above period	$30,450
Less client's income of $185/month for above period (client would have been allowed to keep $25/month for personal needs)	−7,770
Potential Cost would have been	$22,680
Less Cost of MAO Services	−3,346
Savings to Government	$19,334

Case C

Mrs. F.'s condition was diagnosed as arteriosclerotic cerebral vascular disease, and surgery had to be performed to remove plaque deposits. Because her recovery was not as complete nor as fast as she had expected, she became despondent and made arrangements to move to a nursing home, even though she certainly did not want to. After a discussion with a MAO counselor, this client was assured of the supportive services necessary to continue independent living.

Costs if the Client had been Institutionalized
from July, 1975 to December, 1977

Average Basic Cost of Nursing Home Care at $725/month for period above	$21,750
Less client's income of $143/month (client would have been allowed to keep $25/month for personal needs)	−4,860
Potential Cost	$16,890
Less Cost of MAO Services	−3,222
Savings to Government	$13,668

IN-HOME HEALTH SERVICES IN FOREIGN COUNTRIES

In Europe, in-home health services are widely accepted. The two countries which offer the largest volume and broadest range of services, Sweden and the United Kingdom, have faced a growing proportion of elderly and have responded through acknowledging the natural desire of most people to remain in their own homes and the responsibility of society to see to their care. As reported by the Kahanas:[9]

> The proportion of bedfast and functionally impaired individuals living at home is at least as great as the proportion who are institutionalized. In a cross-national study of the health status of elderly people, comparative data were obtained from six industrialized countries, including Denmark, Britain, United States, Poland and Yugoslavia. Although there were some variations among countries, striking similarities were also found, with about 75 percent of the aged population being ambulatory and about 25 percent bedfast, housebound, or able to get around with difficulty. These data suggest a need for careful consideration of alternatives before institutionalization of elderly persons and point to the need for supportive services in the home.

Undoubtedly, the cost advantages of in-home services over institutionalization have been a major factor in motivating the above countries to utilize such programs.

With respect to the 300,000 elderly estimated to be inappropriately placed in nursing homes in the United States, a conservative estimate at the rate of $400 per month for home care vs. $700 per month for institutionalized care would place potential cost reduction at over $1 billion per year. This does not take into account the savings to be derived from not having to expand facilities. Other benefits would be the more optimal provision of services to the expanding elderly population, as well as the sociological and psychological benefits to which a dollar value assignment is impossible.

CAN HOME CARE PREVENT INSTITUTIONALIZATION?

A few localized studies suggest that home care can prevent institutionalization. Using the number of home health starts per 1,000 Medicare beneficiaries as his measure, Dunlop[10] in a multivariate analysis of nursing home utilization, found that increases in home health care were associated with decreases in the utilization of nursing homes and related facilities. In an investigation of 245 patients in a New York City program for the homebound aged, Brickner[11] et al. reported that after 24 months, 23 patients improved to the extent that they were no longer homebound, 116 remained stabilized under the program's continuing care, and 40 patients were in institutions, either in hospitals or nursing homes. Relying solely on clinical judgment, the authors estimated that 85 of the patients would have required institutional care and 25 of the patients would have died without the program.

The most widely cited home care studies concerning cost savings are of short-term, acutely ill patients. Conceptually, any chronically disabled person can be maintained at home if enough resources are expended. Further, it appears reasonable to assume that the cost of services is related to the level of the patient's disability. If this is the case, the problem is to establish some break-even point at which economies of scale in nursing homes make it more expensive to maintain a person at home than in an institution. As Brickner, et al.[12] noted, a program for the homebound in New York City could claim considerable cost savings, but that claim was based solely on physician estimates of "probable" institutionalization. In addition, Brickner et al. estimated only one year savings, not the counterbalancing costs of several years of possible home care maintenance.

In a report to Congress from the Controller General's Office,[13] it was pointed out that until older people become greatly or extremely impaired, the cost for home services, including the large portion provided by families and friends, is less than the cost of putting these people in institutions. About seventeen percent of those 65 years or over fall within the greatly impaired category and about one-third of them are in institutions. For this group, the value of supportive services provided by families and friends becomes so high that home care costs more than that provided by institutions.

Furthermore, as an individual becomes more impaired, the costs or values of home services increase and the proportion of care provided by families and friends also increases. At the "greatly impaired" level where the break-even point in cost is reached, it was reported that families and friends were providing over 70 percent of the value of services received by older people. Families and friends caring for the "greatly impaired" were providing about $287 per month in services for every $120 being spent by agencies.

IMPACT OF MEDICAID AND MEDICARE

Medicare and Medicaid are the driving forces in the formation and implementation of long-term care policies for government. As such, the lack of priority that the United States has given to home health is apparent from the small portion of Medicare and Medicaid expenditures on them, approximately $356 million compared to $5.6 billion for institutional care. Under Medicare, in-home health services are restricted and carry the skilled nursing requirement. Under Medicaid, basic and even preventive care are authorized. Again, however, the policy decisions have stumbled in their implementation through bureaucratic mishandling and misconduct.

Even a policy alternative to institutionalization which is as equitable, dignified and cost-effective as in-home care has not been able to evolve unscathed through the policy formation process. A real question regarding the efficiency of the system should be asked. Or maybe the problem is just that society does not have the moral conviction to see that the issues it raises are solved. Perhaps these are "pseudo issues" rather than failures in policy.

In hopes of alleviating some of the cloudiness that has surrounded the issue and deterred any concerted effort directed toward the establishment of a clear national policy, the New York State legislature, in 1978, passed Senator T. Lombardi's legislation initiating a "nursing home without walls" program. The program's founders reasoned that, although a nursing home is now authorized to care for a certain number of patients within a facility, there is no reason why that same facility could not also provide the same level of care to people in their own homes. The nursing home would manage the patient's case, but the patient would not physically reside in the facility.

A facility applying to the State Health Commissioner for "nursing home without walls" status must make available, either directly or through contract arrangements, the following services: nursing; home health aides; physical, occupational, respiratory and speech therapy; audiology; medical social work; nutritional services; personal care; homemaker and housekeeper services; and medical supplies equipment and appliances. Nursing, home aide, personal care, and homemaker services must be available 24 hours per day, seven days per week. Each provider must have a physician advisory committee with the responsibility of developing and approving standard medical regimens and policies.

Payment for this program has been made under the Medicare program, with the monthly budget limited to 75 percent of the average monthly skilled nursing facility rate. For example, if the average skilled nursing facility rate in a county is $1200 per month, up to $900 per month is available for a "nursing home without walls" patient. If the patient requires health services costing $600, the $300 balance accrues to the account and can be used at a later date if the needs become more costly.

The department of social services has estimated that in its first year of operation, the "nursing home without walls" program resulted in savings of $11.8 million over what it would have had to spend on care for the same patients in residential health care facilities.

CONCLUSIONS

In expanding the financial coverage of home care, caution must be exercised not to open a Pandora's Box. Efforts must be exerted to maintain control over the expansion of services so as not to generate abuses similar to those which have occurred in the nursing home industry. Likewise, programs must be evaluated in terms of equity, dignity and cost. For example, incentives to families or relatives must be developed for providing home care to elderly. Only through efforts such as those by the New York State legislature will a comprehensive long-term care policy incorporating in-home services become a reality.

NOTES

1. *Home Health Care in the United States*, Senate Special Committee on Aging (Washington, D.C.: U.S. Government Printing Office, 1976).

2. "Home Health Services in the United States: A Working Paper on Current Status," *In-Home Services: Toward a National Policy*, Conference Proceedings (Washington, D.C.: U.S. Government Printing Office, 1973), p. 12.

3. *Long Term Care: Actuarial Cost Estimate*, Congressional Budget Office (Washington, D.C.: U.S. Government Printing Office, 1977).

4. E. Kahana and B. Kahana, "Health Care Facilities," in F. U. Steinberg, ed., *Cowdry's: The Care of the Geriatric Patient* (St. Louis, Missouri: C. V. Mosby Company, 1976) pp. 451-482.

5. By inappropriate is meant not only the failure to use existing home health care services when available, but also the failure to establish such services as a viable alternative.

6. Congressional Budget Office, *Long Term Care for the Elderly and Disabled*.

7. E. Kahana and B. Kahana, "Health Care Facilities" pp. 451-482.

8. Annual Report 1977, Minneapolis Age and Opportunity Center, Inc., National Institute on Aging.

9. E. Kahana and B. Kahana p. 472.

10. B. Dunlop, *Determinants of Long Term Care Facility Utilization by the Elderly: An Empirical Analysis* (Washington, D.C.: The Urban Institute, 1976).

11. P. W. Brickner, J. F. Janeski, G. Rich, S. T. Duque, L. Starika, R. LaRocco, T. Flannery and S. Werlin, "Home Maintenance of the Home Bound Aged: A Pilot Program in New York City," *The Gerontologist* 16 (1976): pp. 25-29.

12. Ibid, pp. 25-29.

13. *Home Health—The Need for a National Policy to Better Provide for the Elderly*, Comptroller General's Report to the Congress, December, 1977.

Chapter 6

Home Health Care Programs

Home health care, as an alternative to long-term institutional care, has become a valuable resource in many communities. It provides needed services to many people but especially to those elderly ill who are functionally impaired. Although many of these persons receive needed emotional and physical support from relatives or friends, the professional assistance for health problem treatments and health care therapy is an important ingredient that prevents institutionalization in many cases.

A chronic condition such as arthritis or diabetes can cause functional impairment, but is usually not enough to indicate the need for long-term institutional care. The degree of functional impairment is determined by the elderly person's ability to handle daily activities and moving about without assistance. Elderly who are functionally disabled are often bedridden, need assistance with dressing and bathing, or need help in moving around outside the home. These people are typical candidates for home health care and do not necessarily require institutionalization. Availability or lack of institutional facilities, willingness of family or friends to care for the person, costs of care, the person's reluctance to enter an institution, and availability of home care all are important variables to consider when deciding whether a person should enter an institutional facility. Home health care provides a viable alternative for those elderly for whom institutionalization is not the answer.

Generally, home health care is provided or subsidized through a government program. The programs usually operate under federal, state, or county sponsorship and support. They range from those providing strictly health treatment to those that offer a gamut of home services such as diagnostic health care, therapeutic health care, nutrition, transportation, and recreation.

AN INVENTORY OF HOME HEALTH SERVICES

The Council of Home Health Agencies and Community Health Services define Home Health Services as described below[1]

1. An array of health care services provided to individuals and families in their places of residence or in ambulatory care settings for purposes of preventing disease and promoting, maintaining or restoring health, or minimizing the effects of illness and disability.
2. Services appropriate to the needs of the individual and his family are planned, coordinated and made available by an organized health agency through the use of agency employed staff, contractual arrangements or a combination of administrative patterns. Medical services are primarily provided by the individual's private or clinic physician.

There are currently over 2,000 agencies in this country providing home health services. Unfortunately however, similar to the nation's health care delivery system, there is great disparity from one region to another in the amount and variety of services available. In thinly populated areas, home health services are often minimal or unavailable.

The essential home health services that are often eligible for insurance coverage are listed below. Those services that would normally be arranged by a home health agency and facilitated by patient transportation services are marked with an asterisk.

A. Basic Essential Services
        Home health aide-homemaker
        Medical supplies and equipment
        Nursing
        Nutrition
        Occupational therapy
        Physical therapy
        Speech pathology services
        Social work
B. Other Essential Services
        Audiological services*
        Dental services*
        Home-delivered meals
        Housekeeping services
        Information and referral services
        Laboratory services*
        Ophthalmological services*
        Patient transportation and escort services
        Physicians services*
        Podiatry services*
        Prescription drugs

Prosthetic/orthotic services*
Respiratory therapy services
X-ray services

In addition, there are desirable services that may be obtained through other community support programs designed to help those aged who are well but still dependent. They include:

Barber/cosmetology services
Handyman services
Heavy cleaning services
Legal and protective services
Pastoral services
Personal contact services
Recreation services
Translation services

WHAT HOME HEALTH CARE HOPES TO ACCOMPLISH

The primary objectives of coordinated home care have been summarized by Littauer[2] as listed below:

- to furnish comprehensive medical, nursing, social work, and related care to patients in their homes, whose needs can be satisfactorily met in this milieu.

- to furnish "better" care in the home for selected types of patients than would be possible in the institutions.

- to furnish comprehensive care at lower cost than the institutional setting by using the home for treatment.

- to shorten the hospital stay, or prevent the hospitalization or rehospitalization of selected patients.

- to improve utilization of existing facilities and reduce demand for more beds by releasing hospital beds for those who need them.

- to expedite recovery, prevent or postpone disability, and maintain personal dignity by restoring patients to normal family living and useful functional activity.

Quality home care programs can provide an array of services that satisfy the needs of the homebound elderly. However, many problems have to be solved before home care programs can reach their potential value in relation to the total health care delivery system.

SIZE OF THE HOME HEALTH CARE INDUSTRY

Home health care is still only a fraction of the size of the institutional health care industry. Specifically, home health care accounts for less than 1 percent of Medicare expenditures and only about 0.5 percent of Medicaid expenditures. Since 95 percent of the elderly population are not institutionalized, and 80 percent of that group has some level of impairment, it becomes clear that there is a great potential demand for home health care services.

Lack of coordination and lack of knowledge about available services are generally accepted deficiencies in the health care system. Still the number of agencies providing home health care is growing. In 1975 there were less than 1,800 administrative units providing homemaker services, and fewer than half of these were among the 2,300 certified agencies. In order to provide home services under Medicare, a certified home health agency must provide skilled nursing care plus at least one other service such as physical therapy, speech therapy, occupational therapy, medical social work, or home health aide service. During the mid-1970s the number of homemakers (an important component) was estimated at about 44,000. The National Council of Homemaker-Home Health Aides, the standard-setting body, places the need at 300,000, approximately 1 for every 1,000 Americans under age 65, and 1 to 100 for those 65 and over. Currently the U.S. has 1 homemaker aide for every 5,000 persons, a very low ratio compared with that of other industrialized nations such as Norway, The Netherlands, Sweden, or England. Sweden has the highest ratio, with approximately 1 aide for every 121 persons.[3] Of course, the approach to health care in these countries is different than in the U.S. and foreign health care generally enjoys much greater government support.

COST EFFECTIVENESS AND SOCIAL APPROPRIATENESS OF HOME HEALTH CARE

The cost and cost effectiveness of home health care, including homemaker services, have been debated for some years. Interest in the cost effectiveness of this service stems from the combined pressures of the "geriatric boom," the rising cost of health care, and a concern for overall quality of care for the aged.

A review of the literature to determine under what conditions home health care is both cost-effective and socially appropriate failed to produce an analysis that combined both the social and economic aspects. Interviews with social workers, nursing home administrators, home health agencies, and other health care professionals revealed that home health care is justified from the perspective of need rather than from the perspective of cost-effectiveness. There is a broad range of opinion as to what policies are desirable and possible. What is needed is some consensus in regard to purpose and goals.

There is however, unanimous agreement that two variables—family support and the patient's level of impairment—are the key factors that determine the use of home health care. Whether implicitly or explicitly stated, the availability of family support is central in determining whether home health care services represent a viable alternative to institutionalization.

Despite the continuing willingness of families to support the aged, historical changes have created new constraints on families, and these must be considered in policy decisions.

An abundance of recent literature on intergenerational relationships addresses various aspects of this issue. These findings should be integrated into the cost-effectiveness debate. While the methodology in some of these studies still needs some refinement, the studies do substantiate the need for caution in assuming the continued existence or desirability of extensive family support as suggested in the cost-effectiveness studies.

In fact, it is difficult to determine just what the "true" costs are. According to the Comptroller General's 1977 Government Accounting Office (GAO) Report:[4] "The true costs of maintaining the elderly and sick in their homes have been largely hidden because the greatest portion of such costs represent the services provided by families and friends rather than those provided at public expense." This statement has enormous social and policy implications and suggests that further interdisciplinary research is needed.

It has been suggested that just as the Medicare-Medicaid programs were created as a response to pressures from providers, doctors, and hospitals that were not receiving payment, new approaches to dealing with the "geriatric problem" might well evolve from the pressures of families. Future policy recommendations will reflect the changing needs and attitudes of both the older and the younger segment of the population. In other words, a long-term policy is indicated, and it is unlikely that such a program will be accomplished easily. For the time being, health professionals are stressing the savings potential of home health care in hopes that this emphasis will reveal entirely different approaches to the problem.

According to the 1974 U.S. Senate Subcommittee on Long-Term Care:[5]

> If home health services are readily available prior to placement in a nursing home, there is convincing evidence to conclude that such care may not only postpone but possibly prevent more costly institutionalization. What is particularly appealing from the standpoint of the elderly is that home health services can enable them to live independently in their own homes, where most of them would prefer to be.

This conclusion was reached after 15 years of study of long-term care and after testimony of hundreds of witnesses, both health professionals and consumers.

Other studies support this view and stress the "independence" and "choice" elements. It has been estimated that 85 percent of the elderly, both those in nursing homes and those living independently, prefer home care. This raises the issue of choice, an element generally considered lacking in our present health care delivery system.

THE ELEMENT OF CHOICE

At present, the elderly's choice of health care options is limited and influenced by reimbursement mechanisms. Although choice is an ideal in our democratic society, in reality it is an option only for the affluent. Of course some say that in regard to home health care, individual choice may place unreasonable demands on other segments of the population and may thus infringe on their economic and social freedom. In short the issue of choice has economic, philosophical, and political dimensions.

Home health advocates claim that if home health services are available they would be the choice of many elderly, and the resulting earlier discharges and decrease in admissions would lead to considerable savings. Realistically, however, choice must be combined with an accurate assessment of level of impairment. This other key element has prompted a search for a more adequate way to determine the appropriateness of such services on an individual basis. In some states the responsibility has fallen to hospital utilization review committees. For instance, New York State mandates an organized discharge planning program that must be submitted to the Commissioner of Health in writing "to ensure that each patient has a planned program which meets the patient's postcharge needs." There is some disagreement among health care providers as to the effectiveness of this approach, and administrative problems need to be ironed out. Discharge planners, on the other hand, criticize the lack of coordination and varying quality of home health care and contend that these conditions inhibit their effectiveness.

Unfortunately, as stated previously, choice is not always an option for the dependent elderly in our society. As a result, most of the studies that have compared home health care to nursing home care have addressed the cost issue in considerable detail and have given only token attention to the choice issue. Another drawback of these studies is that they rarely consider the abilities, attitudes, and needs of both the elderly and their families in regard to providing home health care as well as receiving it.

The previously cited 1977 GAO report makes the following recommendations:[6]

> Until older people become greatly or extremely impaired, the cost of
> nursing home care exceeds the cost of home care including the value

of the general support services provided by family and friends. However, for the greatly or extremely impaired, the value of services provided by family and friends becomes a dominant factor in their care and well being. Thus, those greatly or extremely impaired elderly who live alone are the most likely to become institutionalized. The Congress should consider focusing the jobs to be created to assist the sick and elderly under the President's welfare reform proposal to those elderly who live alone and are without family support.

Because the states and HEW are experiencing considerable difficulty in coordinating the many federal programs which offer home health benefits, HEW should develop for the Congress consideration a comprehensive national policy for the delivery of home health services.

This report is a prime example of how misleading and incomplete data can lead to the assumption that expansion of home health care is the universal solution to the problem. In a review of the literature on home health care effectiveness studies, John Hammond[7] points out that our available data are based on existing programs rather than on systematic research designs and rarely includes consideration of direct, indirect, and tangible benefits and costs. And although it has received a great deal of attention in gerontology literature, the concept of the informal support or natural helping network has not been integrated into home health care cost-effectiveness studies.

THE NETWORK CONCEPT OF CARING FOR THE ELDERLY

The network concept is based on the recognition that society is becoming increasingly complex and interrelated and there is a need for correspondingly complex concepts and descriptive analysis. According to Cantor[8] this network includes friends, neighbors, and relatives and functions to enable the elderly person to maintain independent living in the community.

Other studies, like the one reported by Johnson and Bursk,[9] have emphasized the critical significance of the affective relationship between elderly persons and their adult children. Many of these studies have shown that families and friends are indeed involved in providing the daily living requirements of older people, as reported by the GAO. These services include transportation, shopping and financial assistance. However, the question remains: To what extent can the family be expected to assume the burden of long-term care? Often the family provides resources to the point of exhaustion, asking for help only when strained beyond endurance.

A study by Eggert et al.[10] confirms the family's willingness to assume the burden of care for seriously impaired individuals, but also suggests that without supportive services the family's capacity to provide care is fragile. The study found that 70 percent of the patients who were institutionalized had been cared for at home after a previous hospitalization. However, after a second hospitalization, only 38 percent of these families were willing to continue providing care. This breaking point contradicts the break-even point referred to in the GAO cost comparison. The Eggert study suggests that the lack of available support services erodes a family's willingness and capacity to care for an elderly relative who is ill and is responsible for a rise in institutionalization.

Historical and social changes have created new constraints on families. Demographic changes have reduced the number of descendants to whom an older person may turn for assistance. Changes in the economy have decreased a parent's power to ensure support by grown offspring. Various forces acting on the family—social legislation giving individuals more independence, greater mobility, more emphasis within the family on raising children, more mothers working—have distorted the traditional interdependencies between the elderly and their children.

Probably most significant is the change in women's social roles, particularly the fact that at present approximately 60 percent of all women between 18 and 64 are working outside the home. This figure will no doubt increase steadily as the level of education increases. As more and more women work, the opportunity to take care of one's parents declines.

The research into intergenerational relations has obvious implications for policy and planning. The general consensus of findings by Cantor[11] and Shanas and Sussman[12] indicate that the capacities and capabilities of the formal and informal system differ significantly. For instance, with both husband and wife working, the capability of caring for a parent still exists, but the capacity is no longer available. There are also indications that the best situation is one in which families can rely on the "bureaucracy" for assistance with economic and health care while continuing to draw on its own resources to meet the emotional and environmental needs of older people. These studies suggest that policy makers and practitioners should pay greater attention to intervention strategies aimed at improving the correlation between poor health and poor intergeneration relationships.

Supportive services that would strengthen the network concept include improved transportation, home medical services, financial assistance where needed, day care centers, and respite care services. The latter are temporary care services, which give some needed relief to families of the aged, ultimately improve intergenerational relationships, and benefit society as a whole.

The economic approach to the study of home health services can provide administrators and policy makers with valuable information as to the optimal level for delivery and allocation of alternative services. However, the economic approach to planning is tremendously enhanced by sociological and psychological studies. The GAO report mentioned earlier fails to meet this criteria. While many would concur with the GAO that family support is the key element, the recommendations made by this report should not be accepted. Improvement in the management of services must be based on data that is more reliable and more diverse.

CASE STUDY OF A HOME HEALTH CARE PROGRAM

A journal article by Brickner and Scharer[13] describes how home health care is provided through a New York City hospital-based home health care program. The program was started in 1973 by St. Vincent's Hospital to provide professional health services to homebound, isolated, and abandoned elderly people living in Chelsea and Greenwich Village, areas surrounding the hospital. The goals of the program were to keep patients in their own community, out of institutions, in adequate housing, in the best possible state of health, and at the maximum possible level of independence.

During the first four years of the program, 466 individuals participated at various times. Over 3,500 home visits were made. The average age of the patients was 80 years old; two-thirds were women, and two-thirds lived alone. The problems of the patients involved not only physical and mental impairments but also financial, housing, and social isolation concerns.

To provide the needed services, the hospital used a team approach. The team consisted of a coordinator, physician, nurse, and social worker. In certain cases a homemaker participated on the team. Teams saw patients by appointment, arranged by the coordinator. The nurse, physician, and social worker were usually present during home visits. It was found that the health problems of the homebound elderly frequently required both a physician and a nurse, and sometimes also a social worker. Physicians participated on a regular basis because the program was based at a hospital. This meant that the program could tap the hospital's physician pool, even when a subspecialist—such as a psychiatrist, a dermatologist, or an urologist—was needed. If a patient became seriously ill, it was easy to secure access to a hospital bed. A medical file was already available on that patient, thus providing for continuity of care.

The authors argued that although most home health care is provided by free-standing community agencies or agencies whose primary commitment is to homemaker services, it is unlikely that these agencies could serve the elderly as well as a hospital-based home care program similar to the one at St. Vincent's. Because the elderly ill have complex needs, to serve them well, keep them out of institutions, and return them to a satisfactory level of health and independence requires the team approach.

The St. Vincent's program was supported by private grants and to a lesser degree by the New York City Department of Health. Care was provided free of charge to ensure that lack of money did not prevent a patient from requesting or accepting care. Although most patients were covered by Medicare and some also by Medicaid, the hospital employees cannot be reimbursed for home care services. Only hospitals certified under Medicare as home health agencies can bill Medicare for home care services. However, even with certification, only part of the cost of St. Vincent's home care team was reimbursable under Medicare.

The cost of the home care program came to about $105 per visit in 1975 dollars. It was estimated that this cost was about half the cost of institutionalization. Cost comparisons are, however, dependent on many factors. The important benefit of the St. Vincent's program is the fact that many elderly people are now leading independent lives in home settings instead of being institutionalized.

CONCLUSIONS

Home health care services are an important component of the various health care options available to the elderly ill. Although the home health care industry is growing rapidly, it appears that home care will remain a small component of the total health care system for the elderly. Institutional care has been developed more fully and does not depend on the support of relatives, family, and friends to keep the elderly in a home environment.

At present, the most rapidly growing sector of home care is the provision of home health aides and homemaker services. These positions are low paid, and as more and more women join the labor force at increasingly high levels of education, it will become even more difficult to recruit women to provide these services. As a result, home care will suffer.

Nevertheless, home care is here to stay. Those elderly ill who have some measure of network support will continue to have more choice as to the type of care available to them. No longer will they be shunted automatically to a nursing home following hospital treatment for a serious illness. Home care will be available for the fortunate and these people will experience the independence, security, and cheerfulness that comes from living in a home environment.

NOTES

1. Council of Home Health Agencies and Community Health Services, National League for Nursing, N.Y. "Proposed Model for the Delivery of Home Health Services," 1974.

2. D. Littauer, "The Principles and Practices of Home Care," *Selected Papers from the Institute of Coordinated Home Care* (Pittsburgh, Pa.: Institute of Coordinated Home Care, 1963).

3. GAO Report to the Congress, *Home Health—The Need for National Policy to Better Provide for the Elderly,* December 30, 1977.

4. Ibid.

5. U.S. Senate, Subcommittee on Long-Term Care of the Special Committee on Aging, *Nursing Home Care in the U.S.: Failure in Public Policy, Introductory Report*, 93rd Congress, 1974.

6. GAO Report, *Home Health*.

7. J. Hammond, "Home Health Care Cost Effectiveness—An Overview of the Literature," *Public Health Reports* 94, 4 (July–August 1979): 305–311.

8. M. H. Cantor, "Life Space and the Social Support System of the Inner City Elderly of New York," *The Gerontologist* 15 (1975): 23–27.

9. E. S. Johnson and B. J. Bursk, "Relationships Between the Elderly and Their Adult Children," *Gerontologist* 17 (1977): 90–96.

10. G. M. Eggert, C. V. Granger, R. Morris, and S. F. Pendleton, "Caring for the Patient with Long-Term Disability," *Geriatrics* Vol. 32 (October 1977): 102–115.

11. Cantor, "Life Space and the Social Support System," p. 23–27.

12. E. Shanas and M. Sussman, Editors, *Family, Bureaucracy, and the Elderly* (Durham, N.C.: Duke University Press, 1977).

13. P. Brickner and L. K. Scharer, "Hospital Provides Home Care for Elderly at One-Half Nursing Home Cost," *Forum* Vol. 1 (November–December 1977): 6–12.

Chapter 7

Day Health Care Programs

Day care programs for senior adults are far less developed than nursing home care and home health care. However, there are strong indications that day care programs will become increasingly common.

There are two basic reasons for providing day care: (1) to avoid or prevent admittance to a nursing home for any patient who can live at home but needs a variety of health related services for health maintenance and rehabilitation, and (2) to ensure that the elderly frail will enjoy a better quality of life.

Day care programs should not be confused with senior citizen centers that provide companionship, crafts, lectures, subsidized lunches, and referral services. Neither should day care be confused with home health care, which is for those elderly frail who for various reasons are not motivated to leave their homes because of fear or inhibition, or who do not have the physical or emotional drive to participate in normal everyday activities.

Day care emphasizes health maintenance, health promotion, health restoration, and rehabilitation of physical ailments. Services in a day care center are provided by a team of health care providers including physicians, physical therapists, occupational therapists, social workers, nursing personnel, and so on.

MODEL FOR A DAY CARE PROGRAM

A senior adult day care program[1,2] must provide a basic level of service. This includes a bright and protective environment with generous opportunities for socializing with other senior adults and staff members. The basic level of service should also include for each participant one nutritious meal per day, a rest period, social activities, arts and crafts, appropriate exercises, and transportation to and from home. Participants should be ambulatory or able to operate their own wheelchairs. They should not be incontinent and should be able to administer their own medications with a minimum of supervision.

On a secondary level, the day care program should provide personal care services, family and professional counseling, training in the activities of daily living, and rehabilitative therapy. Personal care services include such activities as personal hygiene, taking baths, cutting nails, meal preparation, exercising, and routine health maintenance activities. Family and professional counseling includes help with legal services, bill paying, arranging for the provision of routine services, health education, and other group activities. Activities of daily living are especially important to those senior adults who need assistance after having become disabled. This includes training in the use of crutches, wheel-chairs, and prosthetic devices. Rehabilitative therapy are those treatments provided by physical, occupational, and speech therapists in order to help the disabled senior resume living as normal a life as is possible.

A model program such as the one described above is probably found in a rehabilitation-oriented nursing home or in a hospital-sponsored facility. The purpose of such a program is to return the clients to a normal environment—either living on their own or with close relatives, such as adult children.

CASE STUDY: A DAY CARE PROGRAM

This case study was provided by Pierotte[3] in an article that describes a San Francisco program supported by an HEW research grant. The day care center was housed in a lounge at the Ralph K. Davis Medical Center. Under the terms of the grant, services were to be provided during the day for patients who attended the day care center from one to five days per week and who remained at home at night. Many patients also received home care to ensure that institutionalization was avoided or delayed as long as possible.

Eligibility requirements for admission to the day care program were quite specific. All patients had to meet the following requirements: (1) be Medicare recipients; (2) have one or more illnesses that interfered with socialization, mobility, or independence; (3) require health monitoring; (4) be under a physician's care; and (5) reside in San Francisco. Special efforts were made to make eligible candidates aware of the program to ensure community-wide representation.

The patients that enrolled in the program had a wide range of health disorders. Most were hard of hearing, many required mobility aids, four were blind, six had severe speech impairments, two required constant oxygen, one required tracheotomy care, and one was on renal dialysis. In addition, most had chronic diseases, including diabetes mellitus, hypertension, cardiac disorders, lung disease, cancer, arthritis, and circulatory disorders. They also evidenced various neurological and developmental conditions.

In addition to these physical problems, the patients had problems involving housing, transportation, family relations, finances, and emotional outlook.

These problems often were intensified by depression, pain, poor self-image, lack of ego status, sensory impairment, and faulty perception.

To avoid an institutional feeling in the program, great effort was made to maintain flexibility, considering each patient as an individual, and keep the rules simple and the regulations to a minimum. Staff members wore casual street clothes and used first names. Schedules were as flexible as possible.

Initially, the program goals were broad and general to meet the assumed needs of an unknown population. As individual and group needs became known, the program became more specifically therapeutic, utilizing therapy specialists from the medical center. The primary initial goal for a patient was to improve the patient's total health in order to ensure that he or she could gain maximum benefits from the therapeutic procedures that were provided.

This was accomplished as follows. Medication regimens were reviewed and revised as necessary. Diets were discussed and health teaching was initiated. Podiatry, dental care, and vision and hearing screening were instituted, with follow-up care in the way of eyeglasses, hearing aids, and necessary surgery. A preventive health program was also begun, which included efforts to recognize symptoms of acute illness early enough to avoid hospitalization. A group exercise program was instituted to help patients maintain or improve their levels of mobility. Individual therapy was provided to those who were capable of rehabilitation.

To ensure that patients did not become too dependent on the day care program, it was made clear to them that the objective of the program was eventual discharge. As the program progressed and the patient's conditions improved, a discharge procedure was developed.

The discharge procedure consisted of the following steps: (1) selection of suitable patients for discharge; (2) staff team conference with those patients for identification of discharge needs, referral sources, and goals; (3) conferences with families or caretakers, including social workers, home care coordinators, and involved members of community agencies; (4) a gradual decrease in the number of days per week spent at the day care center; (5) selection of discharge data and criteria for discharge readiness; (6) periodic evaluation of patient readiness; (7) final "graduation" program with gifts, champagne party, pictures, and speeches; (8) follow-up contacts for encouragement, assistance, and information regarding progress; and (9) postgraduate visit to the center to lessen feelings of rejection and to encourage those expecting to leave in the near future.

Although the Davis program eventually had to merge with two other existing area programs because of discontinued federal funding, the benefits provided by the programs and the lessons learned indicate continued and growing support for day care programs. Day care centers are already funded by some states and may eventually become an accepted alternative method of caring for the elderly frail. Without day care, the very ill face institutionalization, and those less ill face isolation and reduced quality of life.

THE COST OF DAY CARE VERSUS THE COST OF NURSING HOME CARE

The following analysis is based on a brief journal article by Grimaldi[4] that commented on a more extensive journal article by Weissert.[5] Weissert's thesis, supported by findings, is that adult day care is less costly than nursing home care. Therefore, Weissert argues, adult day care should be expanded in order to reduce nursing home care. Grimaldi points out several unrealistic assumptions made by Weissert and therefore questions Weissert's conclusion.

Grimaldi argues that during 1975 the average stay in a skilled nursing facility (SNF) was 194 days, and the average stay in an intermediate care facility (ICF) was 249 days. Since Weissert's comparison is based on total annual costs of providing nursing home care versus total annual costs of providing adult day care, the shorter lengths of stay make Weissert's claim invalid. Grimaldi further argues that ICF patients would be more likely candidates for day care than SNF patients, and since ICF per diem costs are generally less than SNF per diem costs, Weissert's case is further weakened.

Grimaldi also argues that estimating the costs of day care is considerably more difficult than estimating the costs of SNF or ICF care. Elaborate statistics are collected and maintained for institutional care, but costs of day care can vary considerably. Furthermore, in estimating the costs of day care, the patient's or patient's relatives' cost to maintain the patient in a home environment is usually not included or is significantly underestimated.

Further, Grimaldi argues that it is unlikely that adult day care centers would furnish all needed medical services. The costs for these additional needed services need to be included in any realistic cost comparison.

Finally, and this is the most disheartening cost fact for advocates of day care centers, an increase in the availability of day care will cause an increase in total number of adults applying for services. People with less severe debilitating problems would normally not be candidates for a nursing home but would take advantage of a day care program in their community. Hence, even if case-by-case costs were comparable, the total expenditures for day care would most certainly be higher.

Therefore one must conclude that on an aggregate cost basis, day care is not necessarily less costly than nursing home care. However, as evident from the description of the San Francisco day care project, the quality of life for many of our elderly can be considerably enhanced by a well-planned and well-managed day care program.

CONCLUSIONS

It is clear from this chapter that day care is probably the most desirable way to enhance the quality of life for many of our frail elderly. In many cases if day care is not available, those elderly in need of such care will either be institutionalized (and suffer the adverse effects inherent in institutionalization) or will remain in a home setting where they will be undertreated and as a result lead miserable lives.

The jury is still out on the cost benefits of day care. One could argue that not offering day care at all would lower overall expenditures. However, in our socially responsible and relatively affluent society we clearly have an obligation to offer day care programs to those elderly frail whose lives would be enhanced by these programs.

NOTES

1. D. M. Morgan, "Day Care as an Alternative to Nursing Homes," *Dimensions in Health Services* (March 1978): 38–39.
2. J. L. C. Dall, "Helping Old People to Continue Living at Home, The Contribution of the Day Hospital," *Royal Society Health Journal* 98, No. 1 (February 1978): 10–11.
3. D. L. Pierotte, "Day Health Care for the Elderly," *Nursing Outlook* 25, No. 8 (August 1977): 519–523.
4. P. L. Grimaldi, "The Costs of Adult Day Care and Nursing Home Care: A Dissenting View," *Inquiry* 16 (Summer 1979): 162–165.
5. W. G. Weissert, "Costs of Adult Day Care: A Comparison to Nursing Homes," *Inquiry* 15 (March 1978): 10–19.

Chapter 8

Assessment and Placement of the Impaired Elderly

Determining who is to receive what service or mixture of services is critical to the allocation of health care resources. This country is slowly recognizing that its wealth is not boundless. If increasing numbers of older Americans are going to have an opportunity to receive the best care that can be offered, their needs must be assessed, matched, and placed with the available services that can best satisfy these needs. The concept of utilization review is implicit within these processes, while assessment and placement activities are necessary as a function of time. Skilled nursing home care may be required during one period of a patient's treatment, but would, hopefully, give way to less intense requirements that could be met through other services such as home care or day care. For this reason, the screening process must be continuous and include periodic review to ensure that the patient is receiving the care prescribed in the most suitable service setting.

If the prime goal of assessment and placement is to fulfill the needs of the patient, it is doubtful that anyone affiliated with those providing these services would be capable of impartial judgment. It is important, therefore, that the process of patient assessment and placement is controlled by an unbiased organization.

PRESENT STATUS OF ASSESSMENT AND PLACEMENT

At present, in most areas of the country, patient assessment is limited to the activities of hospital discharge units that determine the need for continued institutionalization or discharge to a home environment where home or day care can be provided. In the hospital discharge unit, patient assessment is based on medical, functional, and social factors. The patient's physician usually performs the medical evaluation, a registered nurse performs the functional evaluation, and the Social Services Nursing Home Unit handles the social and environmental evaluation. This social and environmental evaluation considers the patient's home environment and ability to return to it. Some patients, after no longer needing acute care hospital services, may require care in a Skilled Nursing Facility (SNF); however, SNF admittance usually results in permanent institutional residence.

Of course, the primary orientation of the hospital discharge unit is to discharge a patient. Because of this natural bias, the discharge unit may make the proper recommendation for that particular time. Still, for the longer term, it may have been better for the patient to have remained in the hospital a while longer and then be discharged to his or her home or to an alternative home care environment.

Similarly, if the person performing assessment and placement is affiliated with a long-term care facility, this may influence the decision in the direction of institutionalization. Despite the enormous increase in the number of nursing home beds, utilization of beds is a still direct function of bed availability. This emphasizes the need for providing an equitable method that allocates nursing home beds to those patients needing them most urgently.

There is another review organization that assesses patients after they have been institutionalized. The medical directors of social services or health departments usually also monitor and review patient placement. However, these reviews are made after the patient has been transferred from the hospital to the nursing home. At that point it is difficult to cancel the placement. Moving patients from a SNF or Health Related Facility (HRF) is extremely difficult because numerous social and political pressures can affect the process. For these reasons the placement or nonplacement decision should be made before institutionalization takes place.

There is yet another problem associated with the assessment activities performed by the hospital discharge unit—namely the variability of quality assessments between hospitals. Remember, the primary function of a hospital discharge unit is to discharge patients. It would seem that a centralized patient assessment procedure (such as shown in Figure 8-1) could minimize variability and guarantee that patient placement recommendations would be made on an equitable basis.

THREE MODELS OF ASSESSMENT AND PLACEMENT

This chapter reviews the experiences of three different urban areas in dealing with the problems of assessment and placement. The three geographic areas that will be reviewed are (1) Erie County in New York State, with its major city of Buffalo; (2) Hamilton, Ontario, Canada; and (3) Monroe County in New York State, with its major city of Rochester. Although assessment and placement activities are heavily oriented towards the potential or present nursing home patient, it should be remembered that noninstitutionalization of a patient

Figure 8-1 Patient Flow Diagram of Preadmission Assessment Process

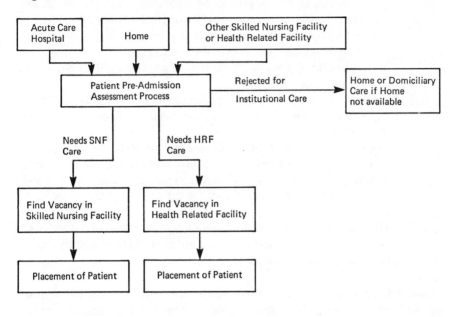

usually implies the need to supply that patient with home health care or day health care, or both.

The Erie County Model

The rising costs of long-term care have been borne by the whole society through a variety of social programs, the major one, of course, being Medicaid. This has motivated an increasing number of government officials to study and develop a process for screening services, a process that could effectively control costs through a more efficient allocation of resources. In September 1975 a report recommending the establishment of a public benefit patient assessment and review corporation was submitted to the Erie County* Health and Human Services Task Force.[1] The report made the following specific recommendations:

   A.   A nursing home patient preadmission assessment and review organization be established:

_____

* Erie County has a population of approximately 1.2 million people and is located in Western New York State.

1. to assess all Medicaid and Medicare patients on a mandatory basis and all private patients on a voluntary basis prior to admission to a Skilled Nursing Facility or Health Related Facility,
2. to set up and operate a bed locator service for SNFs, HRFs, and domiciliary care facilities in the county, and
3. to monitor the utilization reviews of patients in SNFs and HRFs on sampling basis.

B. Recommendations of the organization should be made available to the departments of Health and Social Services and Office for the Aging in the county.
C. The organization be a public benefit organization, established and funded by Erie County with a governing board selected by the county executive. The Board should include representation from the Erie County Health Department, Office for the Aging, and Social Services Department.
D. The staff of the proposed organization should consist of a director or coordinator, a public health nurse, a social worker, a secretary, and a part-time medical consultant.

It was felt that this proposed organization would be highly effective because its single purpose would be to review candidates for nursing homes and to review nursing home patients. It would be an unbiased information source that would not replace any existing county or state control functions. It would simply enable the departments to make better decisions. The report's summary analysis describes the proposed organization's function and status as follows:[2]

> The decisions made by Erie County Departments in response to information supplied by the Patient Assessment and Review Organization would take the form of not approving Medicaid payments when patients are found not to need institutionalized care. In cases where private patients are judged at the preadmission stage not to need institutionalization, a strong recommendation can be made to the affected nursing home not to admit that patient. If these recommendations are ignored consistently the County and State governmental agencies can and should apply considerable pressure on the nursing homes to comply with the recommendations. The N.Y. State Health Department has the legal power to enforce rules requiring that only qualified patients be admitted.

> Therefore, the patient assessment and utilization review organization can only perform evaluations of patients' conditions and report on them to the Erie County Health and Social Services Departments, Of-

fice of the Aging, and N.Y. State Department of Health, to the institutions affected and to the respective patients. Decision making and especially enforcement of the recommendations rests with the Erie County and N.Y. State government agencies.

Certain aspects of the proposed assessment and placement recommendations were implemented eventually, although not through the proposed public benefit nonprofit corporation.

The Hamilton, Ontario Model

It is apparent that many people are involved in the process of patient assessment and utilization review. The patient's personal physician and the hospital planning discharge unit are involved in the patient's transfer from the hospital to a SNF, a HRF, or to a home environment where health care can be provided through home care or day care.

Government agencies come into the picture to evaluate eligibility for Medicaid and Social Service financial assistance. Utilization review necessitates the involvement of the institutional staff or program staff, the physician, and the members of the utilization review committee. Relatives of the patient are bound to become involved. With so many persons concerned with the outcome of placement and assessment, it becomes essential that these activities be performed by an independent organization.

Recognizing the importance of unbiased assessment and placement, the city of Hamilton, in Ontario, Canada, has operated such an organization since 1971. A description of its function, as given in the City's District Health Council annual report of 1974, follows:[3]

> The Assessment and Placement Service (A.P.S.) is a mechanism for ensuring that the needs and assets of people with on-going disabilities are identified, that all facilities and programs that exist to meet such needs are identified, that for each individual the programs or facilities most appropriate to meet his needs is made known to him and professionals caring for him, and that encumbrances to efficient use of these facilities or gaps in services are brought to the attention of the District Health Council, or appropriate authorities with suggestions for remedial action where possible. The A.P.S. is an information generating and exchange system; it does not make the decision on what action to take.

In the Hamilton program, as in the proposed Erie County program, the screening is based on information supplied by physicians (medical), nurses (functional), and social services (social and environmental). The Hamilton Assessment and Placement Unit uses an assessment form that supplies information pertaining to the following categories:

1. *Demographic*—age, sex, marital status, next of kin, education, employment, cultural background, present location, and level of income
2. *Medical*—diagnosis, prognosis, treatment, level of cognitive function, and emotional status
3. *Functional*—degree of ability to walk, talk, see, hear, comprehend, dress, bathe, and undertake personal and household care

The medical information is provided by the applicant's physician. Demographic and functional information is provided by public health nurses and social workers or by the nurse-social worker team of the hospital's discharge unit. An informational flow diagram of the preadmission assessment process is supplied in Figure 8-2.

Monroe County Demonstration Project

In 1970 a demonstration project was established by the Regional Health Planning Council and the Monroe Community Hospital (of Monroe County, New York) to organize a special service for diagnosis, evaluation, and placement of the chronically ill and elderly. The Evaluation and Placement Unit (E-P unit) was staffed by an internist, a public health nurse, and a medical-social worker. Here, too, as in the previously mentioned assessment organizations, patients were accepted for evaluation and placement on referral of physicians, nursing and social agencies, hospital social service departments, family members, and individuals. In addition, a random sample of patients for whom the local Medicaid office had made application for admission to nursing homes were seen in the E-P unit. Of the 332 patients evaluated (from June 1970 to January 1973) for nursing home placement, 22 percent were judged able to remain at home, and only 35 percent were found to need nursing home care. An independent follow-up assessment found that 84 percent of these 332 patients were placed appropriately, a rate 20 percent better than that found in other community studies. The results of the project were stated as follows:[4]

> This demonstrates that a comprehensive evaluation and placement service can achieve significant improvements in the degree of appropriateness of placement of elderly and chronically ill people for long-term care. In addition, it is shown that for many persons for whom admission to nursing homes had been considered the only choice by family or physician, life in their own homes could continue with ap-

Figure 8-2 Information Flow Diagram of Preadmission Assessment Process

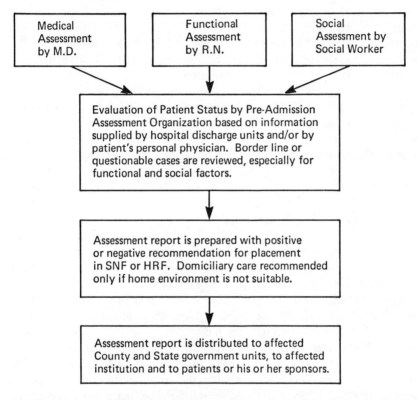

propriate assistance, or life in supervised residential settings more appropriate to their needs and lesser expense could be arranged.

SUMMARY OF THE THREE ASSESSMENT AND PLACEMENT MODELS

The three assessment and placement programs described above are all institution-oriented. This is not surprising since all three grew out of a concern by local government units over the high cost of providing long-term nursing home care. Most of the cost of this care was borne by the public. Providing home or day care was certainly not the main concern of these assessment organizations, because both home and day care were insignificant in relation to the huge resources being devoted to institutional care.

However, all three programs considered the alternative of returning or maintaining a patient in a home environment. What was not always explicitly considered was the need to ensure that home or day care was available. Neither was the patient's choice always explicitly considered, although the social worker's input presumably covered this element.

All three programs were able to evaluate any elderly ill for placement in the appropriate nursing facility or in the appropriate home or day care program. As home and day care becomes increasingly available as an alternative to nursing home care, assessment and placement programs such as the three described above will no doubt expand their activities to do more evaluations of home and day care patients.

THE ISSUE OF TRANSFER TRAUMA

Transfer trauma is a theory that states that change in the environment of an elderly person can cause trauma. This trauma results in higher death and morbidity rates of patients transferred. It is important to consider this issue when outlining the role that independent agencies will play in assessing the elderly presently in long-term care facilities or those about to enter these facilities. Several questions have been raised in the literature: First, are there any possible ill effects to patients that might be caused by transferring a patient to another, more appropriate level of care? (One possibility is transfer trauma.) Second, are transfers to different levels of care within the same facility as beneficial to patients as transfers to other facilities or transfers between a home environment and a long-term care facility? Third, is there some informal or documented procedure by which long-term care facilities can presently manipulate patients' movements through the health care system for their own purposes? And finally, what are the costs involved in all of these situations?

A study was undertaken in Buffalo area nursing homes during Spring 1976. The purpose of the study was to identify patterns of patient flow between levels of care in the health care system. First an exploratory design obtained data on unusual or significant patterns of patient flow and the reasons for such movement. An absorbing Markov model was then used to explore the transfer trauma concept as it applies to elderly nursing home residents. Causal relationships and implications of such transfers were investigated in light of possible assessment and placement activities. A discussion of the actual methodology and technical aspects of the study have been omitted for the sake of simplicity. The remainder of this chapter is devoted to admission of the significance of the findings and the resulting conclusions.[5]

For-Profit versus Nonprofit Nursing Homes

It is important to distinguish some differences between proprietary (for-profit) and nonprofit nursing homes. About 70 percent of all nursing homes are proprietary. These homes tend to have higher turnover rates and have a greater number of private-paying residents. This is simply because New York State, through Medicaid, will not reimburse nursing homes in the amounts they can obtain from private payers. A for-profit nursing home will seek to increase revenue by admitting private payers, and will try to cut its operating costs by attempting to admit healthier patients who need less care. Most of the free-standing facilities—those that provide only one level of care, usually the more intensive and expensive skilled nursing care—are proprietary. Other facilities provide both skilled nursing care and the less intensive health-related or HRF level of care.

Describing Transfer Trauma

A number of investigators have documented an apparent increase in morbidity and mortality rates following a change of residence by elderly people. Other studies have found the evidence to support this theory inconclusive. The most convincing research focuses on differences in morbidity and death after involuntary versus voluntary change of residence.

One may speculate that people's decisions about changes in life status are generally commensurate with their resources. Appropriate decisions are facilitated by the freedom associated with economic independence and with the existence of alternatives. When this freedom of choice is reduced and a person is forced to move out of sheer economic necessity or because of the influence of those in a more dominant position, strain and trauma result. Medicaid and Public Assistance recipients are more prone to involuntary change than is the average person. Simple economics explains this.

Transfers can be described in terms of two kinds of movement—positive and negative. Negative flow is movement from a less intensive level of care to a more intensive level (i.e., from a nursing home to a hospital). Transfers to the same level of care or to a less intensive level are termed positive. Some skeptics of transfer trauma findings suggest that previous data included only those who were being transferred because of a decline in health status. They contend this would automatically bias the conclusions; the patients, when observed after the transfer, would appear to be in worse condition and this would be associated with transfer trauma. These skeptics maintain that in order to be accurate, conclusions about transfer trauma can be drawn only from data that includes positive flow transfers to the same level of care or to less intensive care.

Results of the Transfer Trauma Studies

The results of this study indicate that trauma occurred after inter-facility transfers when patients moved in a positive direction or to the same level of care. The important point is the idea of involuntary change. A Medicaid patient without finances or without someone in the community to provide care has no alternative to the transfer.

Method of payment for care explained some significant differences in patient admission data from the sampled nursing homes. The variable here was where a patient was admitted from. A greater number (45 percent) of those who paid for their own care were admitted from the community. This compares with the 12 percent of Medicaid recipients who were admitted from the community. In both groups, the majority of admissions to nursing homes represent elderly who were living alone. Admissions from a hospital or mental institution were relatively the same for both payment groups. However, a significantly greater percentage of Medicaid patients had been transferred from other nursing homes, 37 percent versus 7.5 percent. Most of these inter-nursing home transfers also resulted in a change in level of care. The majority of patients had been in the more intensive, skilled nursing care (SNF), and after transfer were placed in the lower and less expensive health related care (HRF). This indicates an apparent improvement in health status, or positive flow. In only 15 percent of all interfacility transfers was the flow negative, from HRF to SNF.

The inter-nursing home transferred patients were compared to the nontransfers over a five-month period. They

1. experienced a higher death rate.

2. were more likely to become seriously ill and require a stay in the hospital.

3. were less likely to be discharged home. (In general it was noted that once an elderly person is placed in a nursing home, the likelihood of a discharge is slim.)

Nursing homes that features both levels of care, HRF and SNF, experienced minimal patient movement between levels. No significant trauma appeared to exist after a transfer from one level of care to another within the same facility. Essentially, the social and physical environment remains unchanged in this type of transfer, so there is no traumatic effect.

It is important to note that a majority of the transfers between nursing homes were originally private payers first admitted to proprietary nursing homes. They were transferred after their money ran out and they were forced to seek state aid. As stated before, for-profit nursing homes can make more money from private-pay residents. Since these nursing homes turn over patients faster than nonprofit homes, a hospital wishing to discharge a senior citizen to a less expensive, lower level of care and treatment, will find an open bed faster in a for-profit nursing home. Since a number of these proprietary nursing homes provide only one level of care—that is, skilled nursing care—a patient may be placed in this level of care although his or her condition actually warrants the less expensive HRF care. A hospital discharge unit whose function is to discharge patients as quickly as possible is not necessarily concerned with appropriate placement. If the patient is private paying, the for-profit nursing home is more than willing to accept to its skilled nursing facility an elderly resident who is actually healthy enough to be in a HRF. The state, at this point in time, is indifferent to this kind of inappropriate placement because Medicaid funds are not involved.

After the resident runs out of funds and must go on Medicaid, the nursing home wishes to discharge its obligation. The procedure that follows is simple. The nursing home suggests that the resident has progressed and should be in a lower level of care, HRF. Since the for-profit home may only have skilled nursing care, the resident will have to be transferred to another facility; in many cases this is a nonprofit institution. Transfers to lower levels of care are considered to be good indicators of positive movement through the health care delivery system. The profit motive is always present, but hidden. For-profit homes take credit for efficient, effective management of elderly health care. The state, which is interested in reducing its Medicaid costs, also approves this transfer. The state approves almost any transfer to a less expensive level of care, whether or not it is medically appropriate.

The study suggests there is an increased likelihood of involuntary transfer, such as the one described, and that this results in trauma to the patient. Not only does the individual suffer; the general public also bears the burden of transfer trauma. Increased morbidity means a greater likelihood of yet another transfer—this one to the hospital for a lengthy stay. The costs of hospital care, which are approximately five times that of nursing home care, are reimbursed by Medicaid and ultimately passed on to the public in the form of taxes.

An independent assessment and placement agency would eliminate incorrect initial placement of elderly patients. This would prevent nursing homes from manipulating the care of the aged in order to maximize owner profitability due to changes in patient reimbursement status. An independent agency would also curb the often complacent assessment of patients by state officials who are chiefly interesting in containing Medicaid costs in the short run. Finally, a cost-benefit analysis would prove to the public that an independent assessment and placement agency can be profitable in the long run by reducing the associated costs of transfer trauma.

CONCLUSIONS

This chapter has discussed why patient assessment and review organizations are the best means of allocating our nation's long-term health care resources. Because of the many conflicting pressures faced by hospitals, nursing homes, and physicians to meet their own special interests rather than the patient's, and because society ultimately bears the high costs of institutional care, it is of paramount importance to formulate public policy through which organizations of the type described in this chapter may be formed.

Utilization of acute care hospital beds and SNF and HRF beds is a direct function of bed availability. Faced with an increasing elderly population, it becomes even more important to allocate resources equitably and also limit the quantity of institutions. Needless to say, this institutional service limitation requires the development of alternatives such as home and day care. The Hamilton annual report stated the same problem by saying [6]

> The most crucial defect in the health services at present is the lack of long-term community support programs. Insufficient help is available for individuals who need ongoing supervision to ensure continued optimal function, assistance with housekeeping and home maintenance, involvement in community recreation and vocational activities, and/or sheltered accommodation.

NOTES

1. C. Carl Pegels, "A Report Recommending the Establishment of a Public Benefit Patient Assessment and Review Corporation." (Buffalo, N.Y.: Eric County Health and Human Services Task Force, 1975).

2. Ibid.

3. "Third Annual Report of the Assessment and Placement Service of the Hamilton District Health Council," City of Hamilton, Hamilton, Ontario, Canada; December, 1974.

4. T. F. Williams, J. G. Hill, M. E. Fairbank and K. G. Knox, "Appropriate Placement of the Chronically Ill and Aged," *Journal of the American Medical Association* 226, no. 11 (December 10, 1973): 1335.

5. Paul Gworek, "Elderly Patient Flow and Transfer in the Nursing Home: A Systems Approach," School of Management Working Paper, State University of New York at Buffalo (Spring 1976).

6. "Third Annual Report," City of Hamilton.

Chapter 9

The Nursing Home Industry, The Nursing Home and Its Residents

There are two major reasons why people are in institutions. First, they are likely to be suffering from one or more disabling chronic conditions. Second, they are likely to lack the psychological, social, and/or economic means for dealing with their condition outside an institution. Naturally, it is the elderly that fulfill these requirements more than any other group.

This chapter begins with a discussion of the legal and economic structure of the nursing home industry. The organizational structure of the nursing home and its staff members is examined next. With the passage of the Medicaid and Medicare laws in the 1960s, the nursing home industry mushroomed almost overnight. The rapid growth of the private sector nursing home industry resulted in a shortage of trained administrators. This led to considerable problems for the industry.

Nursing home funding is discussed next. Although many nursing home patients enter a nursing home as patients who are able and willing to pay, the accumulating expenses quickly exhaust life savings, and most nursing home residents end up as public funded patients.

Who is the present nursing home resident? About 5 percent of those over 65 are institutionalized and, as a result, are in little contact with the rest of society. It is important to understand this special population group.

Although the percentage of persons over age 65 keeps rising and is anticipated to continue to climb during the next 50 years, it is unlikely that the actual number of people in institutions will continue to rise at the same rate. This is because there is now increasing pressure to provide alternative forms of care in noninstitutionalized settings.

There will always be a need for the nursing home to provide care for the chronically ill who need constant supervision. This type of nursing home is usually known as a skilled nursing facility (SNF). But what about the many patients in health related facilities (HRFs) and in intermediate care facilities

(ICFs)? Many of these people who can ambulate and are afflicted with relatively minor problems will most likely be cared for in alternative settings in the future.

THE LEGAL AND ECONOMIC STRUCTURE OF THE NURSING HOME INDUSTRY

In order to understand the economic structure of the nursing home industry one must consider the institution itself. Legislation affects not only the services provided for the individual, but also has broad implications for the nursing home industry as a whole.

The nursing home industry has experienced its greatest growth after the enactment of Medicare and Medicaid. Table 9-1 illustrates the dramatic growth of the industry since 1960. Public funds account for about $2 out of every $3 in nursing home revenues. It seems that government, through the enactment of Medicare and Medicaid, has created an industry almost totally dependent upon it. Seventy-seven percent of the nursing homes in the United States are operated for profit, and 67 percent of all nursing home beds are controlled by these homes. Fifteen percent of U.S. nursing homes are philanthropic, accounting for 25 percent of the beds. Eight percent of the homes and beds are government controlled.[1]

ORGANIZATIONAL STRUCTURE OF NURSING HOME INDUSTRY

There are basically two levels of care provided by nursing homes—skilled and intermediate. Skilled care is that level of care nearest to hospital care. Intermediate care facilities, as the name suggests, are intended to help those who do not need round-the-clock nursing care or other mandatory services provided by a skilled nursing home. In some states the term health related facility is used instead of intermediate care facility.

Originally, federal funding under Medicare was available only for skilled nursing care, but in 1967 an amendment to the Social Security Act made possible direct payments to recipients in intermediate care facilities. The law was eventually changed to take the program from its cash grant status under Title 16 of the Social Security Act into Title 19 (Medicaid), thus providing a base for adequate federal regulation.

Based upon the subsequent HEW definitions of the various types of facilities, a 1972 study by the U.S. General Accounting Office revealed that there were 9,244 skilled nursing facilities with 643,403 beds, 4,455 intermediate care facilities with 217,922 beds, and 9,292 related facilities with 238,087

Table 9-1 Estimated Gains in Number of U.S. Nursing Homes, Number of Beds, Employees, and Expenditures for Care, by Percent—1960–1974.

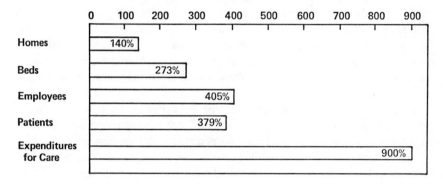

	1960	1970	1974
Homes	9,582	23,000	23,400
Beds	331,000	1,099,412	1,235,404
Employees	100,000	505,031	505,031 (1970)
Patients	290,000	900,000	1,100,000
Expenditures (millions)	$500	$2,827	$4,500

beds. It appears, therefore, that the nursing home industry is evolving into two separate segments: skilled nursing facilities and intermediate care or health–related facilities.

Over half a million people are employed in nursing homes. Their average yearly turnover rate is 60 percent. There are approximately 60 employees for every 100 patients. General and surgical hospitals, by contrast, average 260 employees for every 100 patients.[2]

Studies* indicate that the nursing home administrator, who is responsible for so much, is probably ill-equipped to cope with the demands of the job.[3] About 79 percent have completed high school, and 51 percent have had some training thereafter. Seventy-two percent have no undergraduate or graduate degree, and 65 percent have never taken a course in nursing home administration.

---

* The study cited here is rather dated and the reported statistics may therefore not represent the present. However, the figures do indicate the qualification levels of nursing home administrators.

NURSING HOME FUNDING

As noted previously, the nursing home industry is funded mostly by public monies. Long-term care administered through nursing homes is increasing its share of the nation's health dollar. In 1960 it accounted for a little more than 1 percent, growing to 4 percent in 1970, and to over 5 percent in 1973. In 1972, for the first time, Medicaid expenditures for nursing home care exceeded expenditures for surgical and general hospitals.[4] Nursing homes receive assistance from various government agencies through numerous programs, more than 50 in all.

Because the industry is so dependent on the government, it is quite understandable that industry interests have a significant bearing on policy decisions. Explicit policy enactments, such as laws and regulations that control the quality of care and the proficiency of staff members, are influenced by various components in society that constantly evaluate the system and provide feedback to the policy makers. This dynamic system of evaluation and feedback must consider the effects of any proposed policy on the nursing home industry and the nursing home resident.

WHO ARE THE NURSING HOME RESIDENTS?

Of all persons age 65 and over, 5.6 percent are in institutions. The number of persons 65 and over in the United States has increased 600 percent since the turn of the century. One-third of these people are over 75. Surveys have revealed that only 1 in 18 seniors is in a nursing home or related facility on any given day, but that 1 out of 5 seniors will eventually spend some time in a nursing home.[5]

According to data collected by the National Center for Health Statistics[6], approximately 75 percent of the 1,027,850 persons over 65 living in institutions in 1976 were in nursing homes, 11 percent were in mental hospitals, and 14 percent were in all other types of institutions. Eighty-nine percent of nursing home patients, 28 percent of mental hospital patients, and nearly all residents of geriatric hospitals are over 65.

Because nursing homes supply the bulk of long-term care and because the elderly comprise the greatest proportion of the nursing home population, discussion related to the resident population will be restricted to the nursing home elderly. As pointed out during hearings by the Subcommittee on Long-term Care of the Special Senate Committee on Aging, nursing home patients are generally old, female, widowed, white, and alone, although most are brought into the institution directly from their private homes.[7] Provisional findings of a 1974 HEW "Long-term Care Facility Improvement Study" revealed that of the three thousand SNF patients surveyed, about one out of five were admitted from the community, and four out of five were admitted from another health care facility. The largest proportion of these were admitted from a hospital about 62.5 percent. (This appears reasonable in view of the nature of a SNF.) Senate hearings also disclosed that the average length of stay in a SNF is over two years, and, once entered, a patient usually dies there.

This last fact helps explain the fear and hostility the aged feel about nursing homes. Studies indicate that over 50 percent of patients die in the nursing home.[8] It has been documented that old people believe entry into a home is a prelude to death and that there is a negative relationship between survival and institutionalization.[9]

Disabilities

One of the most common disabilities among nursing home patients is mental illness, affecting more than half of the patients. The second most common disability (as shown in Table 9-2) is circulatory impairment, affecting between one-third and one-half of nursing home patients. About one-quarter of nursing home patients suffer some degree of physical handicap from permanent stiffness. Finally, about 15 percent have a digestive disorder. Nearly 40 percent suffer from four or more chronic disabilities. Nursing home patients do not have isolated disabilities, they have multiple disabilities.

The typical nursing home resident needs many kinds of assistance. Less than half the patients can walk. About 55 percent require assistance in bathing, 47 percent need help in dressing, 11 percent need help in eating, and 33 percent are incontinent.[10] The extent of the care needed is illustrated by HEW's 1974 Skilled Nursing Facility Survey Findings which report that one-third of the 3,437 patients surveyed were totally dependent on nursing staff for their bath. There were 602 patients (17.5 percent) who required spoon feeding. Thirty-one percent of the patients (1,067) did not use the toilet room, and 13.3 percent (457) of the patients could not put on day clothes. While this survey emphasizes the elderly's need for help, it also points out that the aged are not beyond doing some things for themselves.

Demographics

It has been mentioned that institutionalized persons are likely to be old, female, and white. It is also important to remember that they are likely to be poor. Evidence of their poverty is suggested by several factors. First, the elderly generally live on fixed incomes. Furthermore, this income and whatever savings they may have acquired over a lifetime are likely to be diminished in value by inflation. When illness occurs, high medical costs rapidly erode their

Table 9-2 Proportion of Patients with Physical and Mental Disorders and Number of Conditions in Nursing Homes*

Diagnosis and Number of Conditions	Male	Female	All Persons
Diagnosis			
Senility	53%	60%	58%
Mental Illness	20	18	19
Mental Retardation	10	5	7
Glaucoma/Cataracts	9	11	10
Paralysis due to stroke	13	11	11
Paralysis not due to stroke	7	6	6
Arthritis/Rheumatism	26	38	34
Physical deformity	22	24	24
Diabetes	12	14	13
Back disorder	7	11	10
Heart Trouble	32	34	34
All others	6	5	5
Number of Conditions			
No condition	3	1	3
One condition	16	14	15
Two conditions	22	21	21
Three conditions	21	22	22
Four or more	37	40	39

Sources: L.E. Gottesman and E. Hutchinson, "Characteristics of the Institutionalized Elderly," in *A Social Work Guide for Long-Term Care Facilities*, edited by Elaine M. Brody, National Institute of Mental Health (Washington, D.C.: U.S. Government Printing Office, 1974), 27-45.

The National Center for Health Statistics, 1972, 1976, 1977 (Washington, D.C.: U.S. Government Printing Office, 1973, 1977, 1978).

* Entries do not add to 100% due to multiple entries.

financial resources. Finally, when placement in a nursing home is required, the cost of long-term care is apt to be prohibitive. In 1977 average nursing home charges in the United States were about $670 a month[11] (although many SNFs are in excess of 1,000 per month), and in 1976 average Social Security benefits for a retired couple amounted to only $314 a month. Consequently, according to national figures, at least half of the residents in nursing homes are supported by Medicaid or some form of public assistance (see Table 9-3).

Transfers from Mental Institutions

One last characteristic about the institutionalized elderly during the 1970s—an increasing number are discharged mental patients. Thousands of elderly pa-

Table 9-3 Primary Source of Payment in Nursing Homes

Age and Sex	Own Income	Medicare	Medicaid and Other Public Assistance	All Other Sources
Sex				
Male	36%	1%	59%	4%
Female	37	1	60	2
Age				
Under 65 years	18	0.5	76	6
65–74	31	2	64	3
75–84	42	2	53	3
85+	40	1	57	2
Male & Female				
All Ages	37	1	59	3

Source: National Center for Health Statistics (Washington, D.C.: U.S. Government Printing Office, 1975).

tients have been transferred from state mental institutions to nursing homes. Between 1969–73 the number of aged in state mental hospitals decreased 40 percent, from 133,264 to 81,912.[12] This trend is thought to be a result of progressive and innovative thinking intended to reduce patient populations in large and impersonal mental institutions. But another, more important reason may be cost and the desire to substitute federal dollars for state dollars. Unfortunately, the end result is replacement of one inappropriate setting by another.

CONCLUSIONS

The passage of the Medicaid and Medicare laws in the 1960s initiated a period of tremendous expansion for the nursing home industry. As in other industries, too rapid growth led to problems.

As a result there has been extensive government regulation and control to ensure quality care by trained staff members.

Because there has been a movement to deinstitutionalize those elderly with only minor problems, the aged who remain in nursing homes are those chronically ill with severe problems. Their mental and/or physical condition requires constant care and supervision. Whereas age 65 commonly signals passage into senior citizenship, the transition point into acute care nursing homes usually is age 75 or older.

Although home and day care are desirable alternatives for those aged afflicted with minor ailments, there is and always will remain a significant number of elderly who must be cared for in an institution, usually at public expense.

NOTES

1. U.S. General Accounting Office, "Study of Health Facilities Construction Costs," November 28, 1972.
2. U.S. Senate, Subcommittee on Long Term Care of the Special Senate Committee on Aging, "Nursing Home Care in the United States: Failure in Public Policy," November 1974.
3. U.S. Department of Health, Education and Welfare, Public Health Service, Health Resources Administration, N.C.H.S., "Selected Characteristics of Administrators for Nursing and Personal Care Homes: United States, June–August, 1964." Monthly Vital Statistics Report, August 1, 1969.
4. Special Senate Committee on Aging, "Nursing Home Care in the United States."
5. Statistical Abstracts of the United States (Washington, D.C.: U.S. Government Printing Office, 1978), p. 113.
6. National Center for Health Statistics (Washington, D.C.: U.S. Government Printing Office, 1978).
7. Special Senate Committee on Aging, "Nursing Home Care in the United States,"
8. Ibid.
9. L. E. Gottesman and E. Hutchinson, "Characteristics of the Institutionalized Elderly," in *A Social Work Guide for Long-Term Care Facilities*, edited by Elaine M. Brody, National Institute of Mental Health (Washington, D.C.: U.S. Government Printing Office, 1974): 27–45.
10. Special Senate Committee on Aging, "Nursing Home Care in the United States."
11. Statistical Abstracts of the United States, 1978.
12. "Mental Health Care and the Elderly: Shortcomings in Public Policy" Special Committee on Aging, U.S. Congress, November 1973.

Chapter 10

Conditions and Attitudes in Nursing Homes

Senate investigations, public scandals, and muckraking have led to the widespread belief, whether deserved or not, that nursing home care is often abusive, substandard, and extremely expensive. Many nursing home operators have been found guilty of various types of corruption, including fraud and the receiving of kickbacks. Some of the doctors responsible for overseeing patients' health have been accused of shunning their responsibility. Furthermore, nursing home staffs are frequently underpaid, overworked, questionably qualified, and hold attitudes that may be inconsistent with the welfare of the elderly. Despite these inadequacies, the demand for nursing home care continues to rise beyond supply in many areas of the country.

QUALITY CARE AND STANDARDS

Patient abuse in nursing homes has been publicized and well documented. Some extreme examples will serve to emphasize the sometimes deplorable conditions. In 1971 Mrs. Glenda Carlson described her mother's confinement at the Suburban Convalescent Center in South Chicago Heights (Illinois) to the Senate Committee on Long-term Care:[1]

> I visited mother three times weekly, and at unexpected times. Each time, I would purposely look at the right foot . . . Her right foot was purple and black. She screamed with pain if nurses got anywhere near her foot. I was shocked and horrified at the sight and complained that the nurses had not called the physician in to treat mother's right foot . . . Never once did I visit mother when she was diapered. I questioned the nurses as to why a person with my mother's condition of senility, and ulcerated-looking foot, would not be diapered. Their answer was that the administrator of the Convalescent Center did not

approve having diapers on the incontinent patients because it caused too much laundry and cost far too much. Because she wasn't diapered . . . without being aware of it, due to her senility, she would get her hands in her own excrement, scratch the open sores on the right foot and smear it all over herself.

The Suburban Convalescent Center was certified for Medicaid at the time of the hearings.

A letter concerning the plight of a patient at the Carver Convalescent Home in Springfield, Illinois was also entered in the Subcommittee records:

A disability assistance recipient, Mrs. Annie T. Bond, received nursing care in the Carver Convalescent home from October 1965 to February 1968, on which date she transferred to Mary Ann's Nursing Home in Decatur. Mrs. Bond's condition upon admission to Mary Ann's Nursing Home was such that her attending physician and the nursing home staff were quite concerned. Mrs. Bond was covered with decubiti (bedsores) from the waist down. The decubiti on her hips were the size of grapefruits and bones could be seen. The meatus and labia were stuck together with mucous and filth so that tincture of green soap had to be used before a foley catheter could be inserted. Her toes were a solid mass of dirt, stuck together, and not until they had been soaped for three days did the toes come apart.

An investigation of Carver was ordered but never made. The Carver Convalescent Home is no longer in business; it was destroyed in a fire in 1972. Ten patients died. The home was still licensed by the state at the time of the blaze.

These are extreme examples of poor nursing home care, but it is difficult to understand how such homes were ever certified to receive state or federal money. In 1971 a General Accounting Office audit of nursing homes in Oklahoma, New York, and Michigan found that more than half of the homes were violating basic government Medicaid regulations, such as a requirement that patients be visited by a doctor every 30 days. This requirement was completely ignored. The many examples of deficient care cited by investigators underscore the need for federal and state policies that will ensure delivery of quality care in the present nursing home system.

It was the opinion of the Senate Subcommittee on Long-term Care that the 1973 unification of Medicare and Medicaid standards led to the promulgation by HEW of new regulations that eliminated existing standards and substantially lowered requirements for America's nursing homes. (Medicare and Medicaid will be examined more closely later in this book.) However, many experts believe that despite the flaws in the standards, they are sufficiently high to sustain an adequate level of nursing home care if only they were enforced.

There are a variety of reasons why federal and state regulations are not enforced. The reasons cited by the committee centered around variations in state enforcement procedures. The specific reasons were given as follows:[2]

1. Enforcement meant the closure of facilities that were already in short supply, with no place to put the displaced patients.
2. States have few weapons, other than the threat of license revocation, to bring a home into compliance.
3. The license revocation itself was of very little use because of protracted administrative or legal procedures required.
4. Even if the revocation procedure was implemented, judges were reluctant to close a facility when the operator claimed that the deficiencies were being corrected.
5. Nursing home inspections generally are geared to surveying the physical plant rather than assessing the quality of care.

HEW Undersecretary Veneman stated that the "reliance on State enforcement machinery had led to widespread nonenforcement of Federal standards." The same state people who conduct Medicaid and Medicare inspection, using federal criteria, license and inspect homes in accordance with their own state's regulations. This enforcement is further hindered by the fragmentation of responsibility in the regulatory system. A home is licensed and inspected by one agency, paid by a second agency, and assigned residents by a third agency. In most cases, a fourth agency institutes legal proceedings for closure of a home. Such a fragmented system, plagued with such fundamental problems, almost ensures that, regardless of whether standards of quality are met or violated, the home will continue to operate.

ADMINISTRATIVE PRACTICES AND ABUSES

Difficulty in enforcing government standards is not the only issue that stands in the way of developing a practical public policy capable of meeting the requirements of the institutionalized elderly. Unfortunately, the problems are more complex. The tremendous amount of money being poured into these institutions have meant scandal in the form of unethical and illegal administrative practices. Numerous cases of abuse came to light in the early 1970s.

Mary Adelaide Mendelson, a consultant on nursing homes to a Cleveland community planning group, has investigated the nursing home industry extensively. The results of her work appear in the book *Tender Loving Greed*.[3] The book is a condemnation of the practices she encountered in the thousands of homes she investigated. She describes a variety of methods by which nursing home administrators boost health care expenses in order to bilk government agencies. These methods include driving up the expenses of a home artificially through manipulations of ownership; owning ancillary services, such as a pharmacy or a laboratory, for which the home charges itself high prices; or getting a physician to prescribe care that a patient does not need.

One owner of a 30-bed home in Cleveland got his patients to open bank accounts naming himself as custodian. This enabled him to either borrow from his patients' funds as he chose or withdraw fees for unnecessary care. As financial custodian, this nursing home operator could also intercept patients' Social Security pension checks. The few patients who were capable of seeing their own checks were presented with them face down on a clipboard for endorsement.[4]

The issue of drugs is another area wide open to abuse. The average nursing home patient takes 4.4 different drugs per day, some taken two and three times; 70 percent take 5 or more drugs per day.[5] In 1972 drug consumption in nursing homes amounted to 300 million dollars per year. Yet the flow of drugs through these facilities is largely uncontrolled, haphazard, and inefficient.[6] This is certainly inconsistent with any standard of safe care and treatment.

The actual administration and management of the "private" nursing home would normally be of little concern. Certainly, other entrepreneurial businesses operate with little or no government interference. In the context of the Market-Contract economic model, an institution that relied on the voluntary choice of an individual for maintenance of its business would certainly suffer if it provided services of low or inconsistent quality. One would not put a dog in a kennel if the kennel had a reputation for failing to feed or house the animal adequately or if it charged for services not rendered. By this same logic, one would expect that nursing homes giving poor care would go out of business for lack of patients. Unfortunately, there are plenty of patients. So the great amount of government money available for support, and the general apathy by some, has led society to perceive a need for government intervention in the system.

Government involvement in the affairs of business is a complicated subject to which many books have been devoted. The issue goes far beyond the scope of this book. In reality, all levels of government are involved in the operation of nursing homes. As evidenced by the waste, carelessness, and scandal that has been uncovered in many nursing homes, the government agencies that have been responsible for overseeing the efficient and prudent distribution of health care dollars have been doing an inadequate job at best.

SOCIETAL ATTITUDES

The fear and hostility that the elderly feel toward nursing homes is deeply rooted in society's attitudes about death and the value of the aged. Death is feared, denied, and misunderstood by most Americans. It is only natural that the care of those who are dying is administered with something less than enthusiasm. Our laws and conduct reflect the belief that the old have no value. Retirement is almost mandatory at age 65 because our society has decreed that people over 65 are no longer productive or able to make major contributions. It is not surprising that this group of people, who represent 10.8 percent of the total population, commit 25 percent of all reported suicides.[7]

As is sometimes the case, society's attitudes are in opposition. Certain moral and ethical convictions lead to the passage of laws that safeguard the health of those incapable of functioning on their own. But the same society then fails to enforce these laws and turns its back on the elderly for profit. Certainly, any effective public policy must be backed by conviction and the administrative muscle necessary to carry it out.

Society's attitudes toward the elderly are manifest in the very people who are in most intimate contact with them, the nursing home staff. Because it is so important that the nursing home personnel provide quality care, it is useful to explore how the nursing home staff delivers or does not deliver appropriate care.

THE NURSING HOME STAFF

Physician Attitudes

Does the physician provide leadership in the health care system? An excerpt from the Senate Subcommittee's report on long-term care[8] indicates that today's physicians give geriatric care low priority.

Physicians have, to a large degree, shunned the responsibility for personal attention to nursing home patients. One of the reasons for their lack of concern is inadequate training at schools of medicine. Another is the negative attitude toward care of the chronically ill in this nation. Medical directors are needed in U.S. nursing homes. The Subcommittee's May 1974 questionnaire to the 101 U.S. schools of medicine indicates a serious lack of emphasis on geriatrics and long-term care: Eighty-seven percent of the schools indicated that geriatrics was not now a specialty and that they were not contemplating making it one; seventy-four percent of the schools had no program by which students, interns, or residents could fulfill requirements by working in nursing homes; and fifty-three percent stated they had no contact at all with the elderly in nursing homes.

Physicians can do much from their positions of leadership and control, but up to now they have done little. Physicians should be at the forefront of policy changes directed toward improving institutional care; they should lead the way in determining the most effective alternatives. Physicians must take an active role in the care of the elderly. Unless there is a change in physician motivation, either voluntarily or involuntarily, patients will have little opportunity to improve. Certainly physicians carry a large share of responsibility for the scandal of nursing home abuses, but they also have a great potential for improving the nursing home, along with the entire long-term delivery system.

Nursing Staff Attitudes

The findings of the Subcommittee[9] sum up the situation with regard to the nurses, those charged with providing routine care:

Of the 815,000 registered nurses in this nation, only 56,235 are found in nursing homes, and much of their time is devoted to administrative duties. From eighty to ninety percent of the care is provided by more than 280,000 aides and orderlies; a few of them are well trained, but most are literally hired off the streets. Most are grossly overworked and paid at or near the minimum wage. With such working conditions, it is understandable that their turnover rate is seventy-five percent a year.

At present the federal government's staffing ratio standards are extremely low. They require the coverage of only one registered nurse during the day, regardless of the size of the nursing home. By comparison, Connecticut requires one registered nurse for each 30 patients on the day shift, one for every 45 in the evening, and one for each 60 during the night shift.

The registered nurse has an extremely difficult role. She or he oversees much and is responsible for even more due to staffing inadequacies. Ursula and Gerhard Falk write:[10]

She is the inexpensive physician of the nursing home. She is asked by both staff and patients to look at various physical problems of the patients, to diagnose, to treat with and without benefit of a physician and to call for the doctor when she believes an absolute emergency has arisen. She sometimes has the responsibility to employ and supervise aides, orderlies, etc. Since the physician for the most part is unavailable and rarely seen around the home the patient turns for practical solutions and advice to the RN. In the nursing home the nurse has more power and makes more decisions than in a hospital.

The plight of the nurses' aides is similar. They are considered by some to be the most useful, most necessary, and, perhaps, the hardest working of all nursing home staff. Because of their close working relationships with the patients, they are most likely to develop close personal relationships. As mentioned previously, wages are usually minimum, and, like the RN, responsibilities are extreme. Undoubtedly the low pay, difficult work, and inadequate training have contributed to the abuses perpetrated by aides and other nursing personnel.

Certainly the availability of trained personnel is one prerequisite to the formation of any national health policy for the elderly. Unless sufficient numbers of professional people are encouraged to provide the services necessary to sustain adequate care, any policy aimed at ensuring reasonable care for the institutionalized elderly will fail.

Social Worker Attitudes

The nursing home generally has two classes of social workers. The first is a designee whose main function is to report the sociomedical condition of the patient and recommend further disposition. The designee is usually a full-time employee. The education of a designee can range from a high school diploma to a Bachelors degree in any subject. The designee may be responsible for as many as 175 patients. Because employment is provided through the nursing home and because there are plenty of equally qualified people ready to assume the job, the designee holds a tenuous position. Complaints about conditions may lead to dismissal. But the designee has no authority and is powerless to initiate change.

The second class of social workers are social work consultants. They are usually graduates of professional programs and thus much better trained than the typical designee social worker. Their position is similar to that of the designees. They are usually part-time employees of the nursing home, and authority usually rests in the hands of the administrator. A social worker is probably an expense of little value to many administrators. Like the nursing personnel, the social worker is often used inappropriately to suit the monetary needs of the nursing home. If it were not for the legal requirements, the social worker would probably not be included on the staff of many nursing homes.

ILLUSTRATION OF STAFF ATTITUDES

Ursula and Gerhard Falk have conducted a study[11] on the attitudes of nursing home staff toward patients. They investigated two nursing homes. One was a public health-related facility housing 280 patients in a large dormitory on the campus of a state college. This facility was a branch of a larger county home and infirmary. It had no separate administration or staff; it was administered and staffed by the main home and infirmary located in a rural area about 20 miles away. The second home studied was a proprietary home located in a city suburb and housing about 170 patients.

A total of 53 employees were interviewed and asked 28 questions. These questions were intended to measure such factors as:

- Rejection of dissimilarities
- Receptivity to close personal relations
- Sorrow
- Service orientation
- Rigid expectations

The following points summarize the results obtained from the study:

1. *Staff perceptions of the social characteristics of aged patients*—The staff saw the old and sick patients as dependent, like children, deserving and needing care. This implied that the adult nursing home patients lose their adult status to that of infants. Unlike children however, adult dependency was viewed as unacceptable and patients were thought to be able to take care of themselves if they wanted to. The Falks believed that this indicated that our culture views physical disability as something unacceptable and treats it as if it were a deliberate and malicious act that the patient can control at will.

2. *Staff attitudes concerning similarities and dissimilarities of patients as compared with the general population*—Here the results indicated that the staff viewed patients as different from the general population. The nonprofessional personnel saw nursing home patients as dissimilar from other people with greater frequency than did the professionals.

3. *Staff perceptions of patients' expectations concerning staff behavior*— The staff recognized that patients wished to be involved with them, but they exerted considerable effort to avoid such involvement. This was interpreted to mean that the staff needed to protect itself against constant demands for money, time, and affection; the staff cannot dispense these freely because of their own needs and lack of resources. Further questioning bore out the fact that the nursing home's personnel—both professional and nonprofessional—deemed close personal relations with patients unacceptable.

4. *Staff perceptions of attitudes, and sentiments for individuals working with an aged population*—Results of this portion of the survey showed that nursing home employees found it difficult to understand how a pa-

tient can enjoy life, as they are "forgotten souls." The staff was sympathetic to the condition of being a nursing home patient and identified with the position sufficiently to want to avoid becoming a patient themselves. Both professional and nonprofessional personnel viewed the nursing home patient as an object of sympathy.

5. *Staff descriptions of their duties versus patient's expectations*—The employees recognized that it was their duty to meet the needs of the patients and that many patients would rather do things for themselves. At the same time the staff indicated that they felt overburdened by patients' expectations. Some of the respondents believed that patients imposed upon them; they preferred not to be disturbed.

6. *Staff perceptions of aged individuals who are least "appealing" to the staff*—While the staff recognized a certain amount of self-direction by the patients, this was called "stubbornness" and was attributed to "set ideas." The same trait in younger adults is of course praised as determination and strength. However, since nursing home patients are viewed as children, this attribute was interpreted unfavorably and became a source of annoyance. Many staff were able to recognize intellectually that they should like everyone equally, not only those who appear "happy, cheerful and friendly." Nevertheless they found patient resistance very difficult to handle because it disturbed institutional routines. Staff members often feared they will be blamed for not carrying out policies and procedures that patients resisted.

Also mentioned, as previously indicated, the staff felt underpaid and were not attracted to the job for the salary. This feeling was essentially the same for the professional and nonprofessional staff members.

The Falk study is by no means a complete industry-wide representation of nursing home personnel, but it does serve to point out the existence of attitudinal problems. Staff attitudes reflect society's attitudes, and the disposition of the staff toward the elderly is significant because of their role as care providers. If the United States truly desires to provide equitable care for its institutionalized population, there must be effort directed toward the development of incentives to hire, utilize, and promote qualified personnel. Changing attitudes is an extremely difficult task and cannot be legislated. It is a slow, deliberate process that is initiated by a cognizant society desirous of change. Only this kind of turn-around can produce an environment supportive of long-term quality care.

CONCLUSIONS

Political leadership, social and economic leadership, interest groups, and the general public have focused government attention on a broad array of nursing home issues. Various levels and branches of government have responded in a variety of ways—hearings, studies, and new legislation, and rhetoric, insincere promises, and nonenforcement of existing legislation. Society's generally negative attitudes toward the aged have filtered down through the nursing home's staff, physicians, and administrators. This leads one to wonder if there is now or has ever been a national policy directed toward the provision of long-term care.

The history of public policy toward the nursing home industry (and toward health care in general) has been guided by a simple assumption: more money means better care. Beginning in 1935 with the Social Security Act, to recent changes in Medicaid and Medicare coverage, the government has believed that proper care for the elderly could be ensured through grants, subsidies, and loans. The tremendous inadequacies of the system show that this principle is deficient.

Present policy is in a state of flux. The same principle operates, but with additions. We are beginning to recognize that society's health care resources must be distributed in less of an "ad hoc" manner. The major finding of the Senate Subcommittee on Long-term Care (1974) was that "a coherent, constructive, and progressive national policy has not yet been developed to meet the long-term care needs of the elderly."[12] If society is going to care for the growing numbers of elderly in our nation, a better, more efficient system must develop through the policy process.

NOTES

1. U.S. Senate, Special Subcommittee on Aging, "Hearings—Trends in Long Term Care" (Washington, D.C.: U.S. Government Printing Office, 1970-1971-1972).

2. U.S. Senate, Subcommittee on Long Term Care of the Special Senate Committee on Aging, "Nursing Home Care in the United States: Failure in Public Policy," November 1974.

3. M. A. Mendelson, *Tender Loving Greed* (New York: Alfred A. Knopf, 1974), p. 34-52.

4. Ibid., p. 92.

5. A. Cheung, "A Prospective Study of Drug Preparation and Administration in Extended Care Facilities." Paper submitted to Subcommittee on Long Term Care, 1973.

6. "Nursing Home Care in the United States," Subcommittee on Long Term Care, 1974.

7. *Facts of Life and Death,* National Center for Health Statistics (Washington, D.C.: U.S. Government Printing Office, November 1978).

8. "Nursing Home Care in the United States," Subcommittee on Long Term Care, 1974.

9. Ibid.

10. U. and G. Falk, *The Nursing Home Dilemma—Who Cares?* (Buffalo, N.Y.: Private publication, 1974).

11. Ibid.

12. "Nursing Home Care in the United States," Subcommittee on Long Term Care, 1974.

Chapter 11

Medical Direction in Nursing Homes

P rior to the introduction of Medicare and Medicaid, nursing homes generally operated in isolation from the community's health resources. Nursing homes made arrangements, on an individual basis, with consultant health professionals, with physicians for utilization review, and with hospitals for patient transfer agreements. During the pre-Medicare/Medicaid period nursing homes were not usually considered full-fledged members of the functioning community health system.

Following the passage of Medicare and Medicaid, the financing of long-term nursing home care shifted largely from the individual to the government. Government support is always accompanied by government controls and public scrutiny. Organized groups of legislators, providers, families, and guardians of nursing home residents became interested in how nursing home care was provided and whether it met certain minimum criteria.

An example of such concern was expressed in 1965 in the recommendation of the Commission on Chronic Illness, as reported by Latt.[1]

> No single agency in any community can meet all of the complex needs of the long-term patient, yet without some central organization concerned with those needs, gaps and overlaps in long-term care are almost inevitable. The task of such a central agency is formidable because of the wide range in the needs of long-term patients, the multiplicity of ways through which care is financed, conflicting interests and pressures, the existence of outmoded facilities, and other factors. But the formidable nature of the task is matched by the urgency of need in every community.

The Commission also recommended that more attention be paid to general medical care for the long-term patient. Care for the chronically ill cannot be isolated from the total health care effort without potential deterioration of quality of care.

During the balance of the 1960s and into the 1970s, various interest groups became involved in attempting to develop a model or process by which medical care could best be administered. These interest groups included state associations of the American Medical Association, welfare agencies, medical centers, community hospitals, and university-based physician groups. Their recommendations consisted of medical staff equivalent concepts for nursing homes, medical team supervision of care for nursing home patients, community-based medical teams providing services in nursing homes, and medical advisory committees.

These recommendations inspired HEW regulations, effective in 1976, requiring skilled nursing facilities (SNFs) to provide either a physician serving as medical director or to have an organized medical staff. Since most SNFs are relatively small, most opted for the part-time medical director model; the medical staff option was simply not feasible in most situations.

The National Center for Health Services Research (NCHSR) funded a study to investigate medical direction in SNFs. The results of the study were reported in a 1979 publication titled *Medical Direction in Skilled Nursing Facilities*.[2] Much of this chapter is based on that study.

THE NURSING HOME MEDICAL DIRECTOR

Although the federal government did not require nursing homes to have medical directors or medical staffs until 1976, many nursing homes had retained physicians on a part-time basis to provide medical guidance and patient care. These physicians had organized themselves into the Association of Nursing Home Physicians. The first national meeting of the association was held in Baltimore, Maryland in 1967. A constitution outlining the purposes of the association was adopted at that meeting. As reported by Latt,[3] the purposes included:

> To further the general health of the chronically ill and/or aged through the acquisition, dissemination and exchange of useful and accurate knowledge regarding the medical management and treatment of such individuals, and to undertake in their interest such activities as will improve the welfare of these people. To these ends it is the purpose of the Association to permit and encourage similar local and state associations to become affiliated with it, and to promote among physicians the free exchange of knowledge in respect to this subject; to improve the standards of treatment of nursing home residents, to develop methods of medical care acceptable to the Association.

The association worked diligently in subsequent years to develop the concept of medical direction, the role of medical director, and the physician's role in relationship to the nursing home administrator and the nursing home staff.

Early in 1972 the medical director concept was accepted by several national groups as an important step toward improving the quality of nursing home care. At the same time, unification of Medicare and Medicaid standards for skilled nursing care led to the development of new regulations requiring SNFs to have either a medical director or an organized medical staff. The regulations were not finalized until the end of 1974 and did not become effective until January 1976.[4]

There is by no means unanimous support for the concept of medical director in SNF. Professionals generally agree, however, that directors who fulfill their responsibilities do improve the quality of care rendered. The NCHSR study[5] investigated this contention.

MODELS FOR MEDICAL DIRECTION IN SKILLED NURSING FACILITIES

The NCHSR study identified four models of arrangements for the provision of medical direction in SNFs. The four models consist of:

A. One medical director—one facility
B. One medical director—several facilities
C. Multiple medical directors—one facility
D. Multiple medical directors—several facilities.

The model selected by a skilled nursing facility depends on several factors, including:

● the needs of the facility

● the resources within the facility

● the resources within the community

● an appraisal of the options available.

It is useful to consider a typical facility for each of the four models described in the NCHSR study. These four models have a common dual purpose—to ensure the provision of quality care in a professional environment and to provide medical direction in a SNF.

Typical Facility—Model A

This model is represented by a facility located in a rural community with limited physician resources. A medical director attends 95 percent of the patients in the facility, and there is only one other physician providing care. The facility is dominated by an administrator who has long experience in acute care administration and uses a highly structured approach to the delivery of care. This includes the provision of care by the house physician/medical director who makes rounds regularly and has substantial committee involvement.

Typical Facility—Model B

This model is represented by a facility that has a medical director who spends one day per month in the SNF because he or she lives 80 miles away. The medical director functions in that capacity for four facilities and, in addition, has a part-time practice. This type of arrangement results in problems for both the medical director and the facility. The medical director's availability to the SNF is limited, and medically-related problems must be dealt with only on the day he or she is in the facility.

Typical Facility—Model C

This model is based on a small SNF located in a rural community served by only four physicians. This type of facility may have difficulty recruiting a physician to assume the position of medical director on a permanent basis. Since all four physicians at one time or other provide services to patients in the facility, they may each agree to serve as medical director for a one-year term on a rotating basis. Limited facility funds for medical direction restricts both the number and quality of medical direction functions that are performed. Where the facility administrator has limited managerial or health care institution experience, the medical director may serve in this capacity, relating primarily to the director of nursing. In addition, the medical director may perform some administrative functions such as goal setting, choosing methods for implementation of programs, designing medical records, and evaluating the need for in-service programs.

Typical Facility—Model D

This model describes the case where ten SNFs are operated by a parent corporation. A facility may systematically provide for medical direction by contracting with physicians organized in a large multispecialty group practice. This group assigns a number of physicians to actually perform medical direction in individual facilities. This fundamental arrangement provides an essentially inexhaustible source of medical directors and has the additional advantage of quality control and medical direction development in both the facility and the group practice. This advantage is further promoted by practice of appointing a Coordinating Medical Director whose task is to: (1) organize a medical director group that ensures regular communication among the several medical directors for the purpose of defining their respective roles, (2) monitor their performance, (3) specialize in medical matters encountered in the individual facilities, and (4) act as resource for the standardization of medical and administrative policy.

BARRIERS TO IMPLEMENTATION OF THE MEDICAL DIRECTOR CONCEPT

When the change was made from no requirement for medical direction in a SNF to a mandated requirement, there was bound to be some opposition on the part of the nursing home staff. Nursing homes that had functioned without medical directors quite often had directors of nursing and in some cases administrators fulfilling the tasks typically provided by a medical director. The NCHSR study found that half of the directors of nursing surveyed reported high involvement in six medical direction functions. It was found that medical direction functions were frequently shared between the medical director and other nursing home staff. Rarely were medical direction functions performed exclusively by the individual physician functioning as medical director.

The reluctance of physicians to become medical directors should also be considered. The remuneration for medical director is typically about $500 per month (1978 dollars), for approximately 10 hours of work per week. Based on a physician's average income, the position of medical director is by no means lucrative. Several other issues also inhibit participation:

- reluctance of qualified physicians to assume the role

- confusion concerning the actual role of the medical director

- excessive paper work

- inadequate remuneration

- limited amount of available time for medical direction.

A final barrier, probably the most inhibiting one to a physician (especially a physician in a smaller community), is the need to monitor the quality of care provided to SNF patients. While liaison and education functions are quite straightforward and routine, monitoring patient care usually involves confrontation and possibly criticism of colleagues and peers.

As a result, it is difficult to recruit medical directors for SNFs. When physicians accept these positions, it is usually with the understanding that the position is undertaken as a community responsibility and is not necessarily viewed as a source of additional income. This is borne out by the fact that fully 10 percent of the facilities surveyed in the NCHSR study had volunteer medical directors who served without a fee. These facilities were generally of the nonprofit variety.

BENEFITS OF MEDICAL DIRECTION IN SKILLED NURSING FACILITIES

The major advantages of medical direction as identified by SNF administrators and as reported in the NCHSR study are:

1. the potential ability of the medical director to communicate with and influence physicians to provide better patient care and to interact more effectively with the administrative, nursing, and other facility personnel;
2. the availability of a single medical consultant with whom administrators, nurses, and other staff can discuss specific problems;
3. the improvement in the medical climate and image of the facility both within the community and within the local health professions, thus aiding the professional staff recruitment process; and
4. to provide an important backup in emergencies and in cases where the attending physician fails to respond to the needs of patients.

Having a medical director on board also provides a simple coordinator of the numerous medical direction functions that previously had been performed by various individuals within the SNF.

HOW HEALTH PROFESSIONALS VIEW THE ROLE OF MEDICAL DIRECTOR

Following the HEW requirement (which became effective January 2, 1976) that skilled nursing facilities have a medical director or a medical staff, the AMA in cooperation with various state medical societies organized seminars on medical direction. A total of 29 seminars were held. A questionnaire survey was conducted at most of these seminars. The results of this survey were reported by Ingman et al.[6]

Questionnaires were distributed to attendees at 17 of the 29 seminars. The 17 seminars had a total attendance of about 2,900 people. Completed questionnaires were returned by 47 percent of the participants. Nurses had a 70 percent return rate, physicians had a 50 percent return rate, and administrators had only a 36 percent return rate. About half of the nurses held the position of director of nursing; the balance were administrators or owners of nursing homes.

A majority of the respondents felt that the medical director should primarily be responsible for:

1. creating written policies for physician care
2. enforcing medical staff compliance
3. participating in staff conferences
4. contributing to the quality assurance program.

Many respondents were reluctant to see the medical director conducting floor rounds—a necessary activity for concurrent review of the quality of care. They were also reluctant to assign to the medical director the functions of passing medical opinion on patient applicants, counseling relatives, or providing substitute forms of direct physician care.

In general it can be stated that the study showed that nurses, administrators, and physicians were better able to agree on the bureaucratic functions of the medical director than on functions that might be considered more clinical or activist.

CONCLUSIONS

Today medical direction in SNFs is a fact of life. However, the functions of the medical director are still evolving and will continue to do so for the foreseeable future.

The typical patient in the SNF is not considered clinically challenging by the typical physician. In the Ingman survey only 10 percent of physicians considered that clinical skills were more important than a sympathetic regard for patients.[7] This probably indicates that the SNF patient is viewed as one who needs maintenance care as opposed to rehabilitative care. This means that the position of medical director will not be viewed as challenging by the rehabilitation-oriented physician.

NOTES

1. B. Latt, "The Greater Neglect: Administrative Medicine in the Long-Term Care Facility," *The Medical Director in the Long-Term Care Facility* (American Medical Association, 1977), p. 74–77.

2. National Center for Health Services Research, *Medical Direction in Skilled Nursing Facilities*, Research Summary Series, DHEW Publication No. (PHS) 79-3223 (August 1979), p. 32–46.

3. Latt, "The Great Neglect," p. 74–77.

4. *Federal Register* 39, no. 193 (October 3, 1974) p. 35778.

5. NCHSR, *Medical Direction in Skilled Nursing Facilities*, p. 47.

6. S. R. Ingman, I. R. Lawson, and D. Carboni, "Medical Direction in Long-Term Care," *Journal of the American Geriatrics Society* 26, no. 4 (1978), p. 157–167.

7. Ibid., p. 157–167.

Chapter 12

The Physician Extender in the Nursing Home

The Senate Subcommittee on Long-Term Care[1] provided documentation that physicians do not adequately monitor the conditions of the geriatric patients in nursing homes and, in fact, in many cases avoid visiting their patients regularly.

The reasons for this are many-fold, but several reasons in particular stand out: (1) negative attitudes towards the chronically ill, (2) inadequate medical school training in geriatric care, (3) low third party reimbursement, and (4) the assumption that in the event of major medical problems, the nursing home staff will notify the physician. It should be noted that the Senate hearings were held prior to the effective date that required skilled nursing facilities (SNFs) have medical direction, as outlined in Chapter 11. Hence, at least some of these reasons may no longer be valid.

This chapter explores the feasibility of using physician extenders, such as physician assistants and nurse practitioners, in the SNF. Much of what the physician does in evaluating and caring for SNF patients is of a routine and repetitious nature. Many tasks—such as taking a patient history and giving a physical examination—and many diagnostic and therapeutic procedures can just as well be performed by specially trained physician extenders. In the long-term care facility the most difficult management problem is ensuring the necessary patient coverage by attending physicians. As physician extenders, the physician assistant and the nurse practitioner are trained to perform certain specific delegatable tasks.

Between now and the year 2000, the number of people age 65 and over are projected to increase by about 100 percent. Their use of health care services on a per capita basis is expected to increase by 50 percent. However, the number of physicians willing to meet the medical needs of the elderly is diminishing because of the expanding demands of acute care, insufficient reimbursement, and a sense of frustration with the chronic health problems of the elderly.

Although the physician occupies the center stage in health care, 80 to 90 percent of the care delivered to residents of nursing homes is provided by nurses aides and orderlies. Given the low wage levels, poor working conditions, and minimal opportunities for advancement, these employees have little incentive for providing for this much needed service. As a result, nursing home employees have an annual turnover rate estimated at 75 percent.

ROLE OF THE PHYSICIAN EXTENDER

Although most nurses lack specific training in geriatric nursing, the nurse is the health professional most likely to interact with the patient. But constant attendance to the welfare and comfort of elderly patients may be psychologically and physically draining to those not specifically trained or prepared to deliver this type of care. The physician extender may provide the answer to improving the overall quality of nursing home care.

Nursing home personnel have responded enthusiastically to roles adopted by the physician extender. The physician extender has been identified as a resource person who assists staff in crisis situations, plans health management for patients with complex problems, and acts as a support person for staff members working with terminally ill patients. The physician extender's main function in this setting is to enhance the physician's activity, not to substitute for the physician. By monitoring any abnormal or unusual findings, the physician extender conserves the physician's time.

For the institutionalized patients, the presence of a physician extender means that their problems and needs are most apt to be identified and dealt with immediately by members of the nursing staff and by the physician. The physician extender may improve communications by serving as an available resource, by answering questions, and thus meeting any significant psychological needs of the patient and/or the patient's family.

The role of the physician extender in the long-term nursing facility may be aptly described by the term "supernurse." The physician extender can be expected to spend far more time listening to patient's problems and answering their practical questions than does the busy physician. The physician extender may also bring solace to patients and their families by being trained to treat and discuss death in an open and honest manner.

Although there is great potential for the physician extender in this setting, expectations are not always met. Graduate physician extenders trained in the area of gerontology have described four problem areas: (1) conflict between an administrative and a clinical role, (2) insufficient third party reimbursement to cover the cost of the expanded nursing role in nursing homes, (3) lack of a collaborative role in the health team, and (4) the frustration of working with patients who cannot progress.

Although the first three problems exist in most clinical settings, the fourth problem is one that is peculiar to nursing homes. Generally physicians do not have time to become emotionally involved with their patients, and the aides and orderlies who attend to the patients' needs most frequently treat them in a detached and callous way. This leaves the physician extender as the staffer who can be expected to take extra time to deal with the frustrations indigenous to the nursing home patient.

The Physician Assistant

The physician assistant (PA) is a new health care professional formally trained to function as a health provider. Under supervision of a physician, the PA performs diagnostic and therapeutic management of patients. As of mid-1978, there were over 60 physician assistant programs in the United States. Graduates of these programs are trained to work in such settings as single and multispecialty group practices, health maintenance organizations, community-based public clinics, hospital emergency rooms, hospital operating rooms, and in other hospital settings.[2]

The AMA's Council of Health Manpower, in cooperation with the National Board of Medical Examiners, has developed a national program to certify on the basis of a proficiency examination physician assistants trained in primary care. In addition, the AMA's Council on Medical Education accredits PA education programs.

Most states have enacted legislation to define the scope of practice for the PA. In general, PAs must work under supervision of a physician. Supervision is, however, frequently loosely defined. Along with this legislation most states have also established rules and regulations that define educational requirements for the PA.

Despite these guidelines, the role of the PA is not well defined. How do the duties of the PA relate to those traditionally performed by the nurse and the physician? Because the PA is performing a pioneering function, it may take considerable time to find a suitable way to define and evaluate the PA's role. But since the area of geriatric care is considered to be underserved, it seems to be an area where the PA has the potential to develop into a necessary and valuable source of patient care.

It is useful to examine a typical training program for PAs interested in geriatric care. Becker[3] describes a two-week geriatric internship program for 71 PA students and graduate PAs at the Jewish Institute for Geriatric Care. The goal of the program was to expose the PA student to geriatric medicine and to the medical services of a voluntary long-term care facility dedicated to treating the geriatric patient with rehabilitative and restorative therapies. The program offered the student firsthand experience through assignment to an attending geriatrician. The PAs accompanied physicians on rounds. The physicians provided didactic instruction on problematic diseases and assigned students to independent patient evaluations.

Throughout this two-week period, the PAs were rotated through the cardiology, dentistry, ophthalmology, physical medicine and rehabilitation, podiatry, psychiatry, and radiology services. The purpose of this exposure was to give students an appreciation of the special aspects of these disciplines as they relate to the geriatric patient.

The potential for making the PA the major primary care provider in the SNF is hindered by the issue of staff acceptance. It may be somewhat easier for the nurse practitioner (NP) to function in this role. This is because the NP, especially when viewed as a supernurse, fits into the SNF environment somewhat easier. The next section explores the NP role.

The Nurse Practitioner

It has long been argued that expanding the role of the nurse to provide primary care could alleviate the physician workload and thus improve the supply and quality of primary care. Certainly in many ambulatory care settings nurses have long functioned in this capacity under a physician's supervision. However, the nurse's role as primary care practitioner has never really been accepted by the nurse or by the physician until the development of training programs for nurse practitioners. Nowadays, nurse practitioner programs are quite common at most major universities, and the nurse practitioner of the future will undoubtedly carry a considerable amount of the primary care burden in both institutional and ambulatory settings.

One training program for nurse practitioners in nursing homes has been conducted at the University of Minnesota, as reported by Richard and Miedema.[4] To prepare nurses for an expanded role in primary health care, this certificate program in adult and geriatric health instructs them in:

- systematic collection of data

- identification of normal and abnormal physical and psychosocial findings

- analysis of data to make clinical judgments

- development of a collaborative role with a physician in planning care

- teaching and counseling of patients and family

- utilizing resources in the community.

The six-month program is divided into a didactic portion that is developed jointly by physicians and nurses, and a clinical experience portion that is obtained in ambulatory care facilities. Nursing home personnel have responded positively to graduate nurse practitioners. When questioned, they identified the nurse practitioner as a resource person who assisted in crisis situations, planned health management for patients with complex problems, and acted as a support person for staff members working with terminally ill patients.

NURSE PRACTITIONERS PRACTICING IN A NURSING HOME

McCormick[5] reported on the case of a nurse practitioner who functioned successfully in a nursing home setting. In an attempt to solve the difficult problem of providing high-quality medical care for the aged, a medical nurse practitioner from Park Ridge Hospital (Rochester, New York) was assigned to work with the SNF physician group. To enhance the physician's activity the NP saw all new patients and completed an initial workup that included a preadmission evaluation, a history, and a physical examination. The NP also evaluated the results of the laboratory studies that he/or she ordered, made recommendations, and responded to emergency calls.

Some of the NP's most significant accomplishments, as outlined by the author, included:

1. serving as an available reference person who could answer questions and thus meet significant psychological needs of the patient and the patient's family
2. fulfilling the statutory requirements without unnecessarily overburdening any one physician or taxing the financial status of the facility
3. making better use of the institution's facilities, as evidenced by the ability to treat patients in the SNF rather than having to transfer them to an acute care facility
4. improving the overall quality of nursing care, attributable to the informal teaching role that frequently evolves between nursing staff members and the nurse practitioner.

Another case, reported by Richard and Miedema,[6] describes a nurse who has implemented the NP role in an 87-bed SNF in a rural area. In this setting, nursing home administrators reported an increased number of visits by physicians when patient care responsibilities were shared by the NP-physician team. The authors also reported that NP-physician teams have been instrumental in early detection of illness and have reduced the need for transferring patients to acute care hospitals.

CONCLUSIONS

Because physicians are too frequently disinterested in providing routine care to nursing home patients, it has been advocated to make more and better use of the physician extender.

This chapter has addressed the problems and opportunities associated with using physician extenders—physician assistants and nurse practitioners—in the nursing home setting. Research has shown that physician extenders can function successfully in this setting and provide excellent substitute physician care.

It appears that with the increasing numbers of physician assistants and nurse practitioners, the bulk of routine physician care could well be provided by this group of health professionals.

NOTES

1. U.S. Senate Subcommittee on Long-Term Care, "Doctors in Nursing Homes: Shunned Responsibility," *Nursing Home Care in the United States: Failure in Public Policy,* Supporting Paper 3 (Washington, D.C.: U.S. Government Printing Office, 1975).

2. "Profile of Physician Assistant Profession, 1978, and Profile of Physician Assistant Students, 1978" (Arlington, Virginia: Association of Physician Assistant Programs, 1979), p. 8-12.

3. R. G. Becker, "The Physician Assistant in Geriatric Long-Term Care," *The Gerontologist* 16, no. 4 (1976): 318-21.

4. E. C. Richard and L. Miedema, "The Nurse Practitioner in the Nursing Home," *Journal of Nursing Administration* (March 1977): 11-13.

5. T. R. McCormick, "The Medical Nurse Practitioner in the Skilled Care Facility," *Hospitals, JAHA,* 50, no. 4 (1976): 176-81.

6. Richard and Miedema, "The Nurse Practitioner in the Nursing Home," p. 11-13.

Chapter 13

Regulations and Controls for Nursing Homes

Public financial support is usually accompanied by control and regulation. With passage of Medicare and Medicaid in the Sixties, government at both the federal and state levels became increasingly concerned with the way the public health care dollar was being spent.

One of the first regulations focused on the provision of adequate medical care, this concern eventually evolved into specific care requirements that affected everything from the physical facility to the proficiency of employees in nursing homes.

THE LAW AND REGULATION

Medicare, Title 18 of the Social Security Act, financed through the Social Security System, pays primarily for hospital expenses connected with acute illnesses. In nursing homes, Medicare pays for 100 days of posthospital care. Medicare outlays in nursing homes totaled approximately $340 million in 1968. By 1970 administrative costcutting had reduced expenditures to $180 million. In 1973 they were at $188 million, with approximately seventy thousand out of over one million institutionalized elderly receiving Medicare assistance. By the end of 1977 Medicare expenditures for nursing homes had increased to $362 million.[1] However, the largest portion of society's nursing home expenses has been covered by Medicaid.

Medicaid, Title 19 of the Social Security Act, is the state and federal matching program for the "medically indigent." It pays for long-term care as well as for hospital treatment. Rules for Medicaid eligibility vary considerably from state to state. In some states, especially in the South, people are not eligible for Medicaid if they have any financial assets. Other states allow the elderly to keep a small savings account and still receive Medicaid. Medicaid payments go directly to the institutions that house eligible patients, not to the individuals. In

1972 for the first time Medicaid expenditures for nursing home care exceeded payments to general and surgical hospitals: $1.6 billion as compared to $1.5 billion.[2]

The role played by Medicare and Medicaid in promoting the growth of the proprietary nursing home has been noted previously. These two amendments to the Social Security Act have had greater impact on the health care of the nation's elderly than have any other laws. The two amendments have been modified several times since their passage in 1965. One of the modifications, described earlier, was to change Medicaid coverage to include those patients in skilled nursing facilities. This change in itself has been a major impetus to the growth of the nursing home industry. Because the Medicare and Medicaid laws are responsible for the spending of such large sums of money to a growing segment of our population, and because they have become an integral part of society's health delivery system, public health care policy has revolved and will no doubt continue to revolve around them.

State statutes governing nursing home care and management are being scrutinized throughout the country. In New York State, Governor Carey appointed the Moreland Act Commission to investigate residential care facilities and recommend legislation to improve their standards of care and fiscal accountability. The commission's recommendations formed the basis of 10 new laws signed by the governor. All but one of the new laws amended the state's existing public health laws. One law requires that nursing homes give each patient a copy of a statement of their rights and responsibilities, including their right to adequate medical care, courteous and respectful treatment, and the presentation of grievances. Another one of New York's new laws empowers patients, acting individually or as a class, to sue for damages for deprivation of rights. Where deprivation is found to be willful or in reckless disregard of the rights of the patient, punitive damages may also be assessed. The trend in law is for tighter control of nursing home operations in order to guarantee that patients receive "adequate" care.

Actually, state and federal laws that empower agencies to promulgate "adequate" standards for the regulation and evaluation of nursing homes have existed for several years. But though standards had been set, they had not been enforced. Mary Mendelson writes:[3]

> Again and again, regulators have said that once they were armed with new legislation they would be able to move swiftly and effectively against nursing home abuses. In the past ten years, new laws have been passed, new regulations have been changed. Yet, fundamentally, nothing has changed. Many abuses have long been illegal under various state laws—and it is only too likely that so long as enforce-

ment continues to lag far behind legislation, the new laws, like the old, will merely create the illusion of progress without its substance.

The policy-making process may generate enactments designed to address the issues before it. But without provisions for following through, without implementation, the process will not produce policies that can reconcile the underlying problems.

STATE VERSUS FEDERAL CONTROL

A legal issue at the crux of the nursing home controversy involves the constitutional powers of the federal government over the states. The outpouring of federal tax revenues through Medicare and Medicaid has given the federal government real control by stipulating what qualifications an institution must meet in order to receive assistance. But just how far does this control go?

As we have seen, the administrator has an important role in the operation of a nursing home. In 1965 the Subcommittee on Long-term Care[4] found that large numbers of nursing home administrators were untrained. Moreover, licensure requirements varied greatly among the states; some states had no requirements whatsoever. Samuel Levy, Director of the Massachusetts State Nursing Home Licensure Program, reported that only 18 percent of nursing home administrators had completed college; 25 percent supervised all personnel, and 56 percent supervised nursing care directly. As a result, Senator Edward Kennedy introduced legislation to require states to license nursing home administrators. It stipulated that a State Licensing Board be formed to oversee the licensure process and that the boards must include "representative of professions and insitutations concerned with the care of the chronically ill and the infirm aged patients."[5]

Nursing home administrators sought wide representation on these boards and actually came to dominate them in 24 states. The Nursing Home Association contended that this is entirely consistent with the predominance of physicians, pharmacists, attorneys, and dentists on their own state licensure boards. Congress felt otherwise, and in May 1972 HEW announced regulations requiring representation by all health professionals on the boards; no one profession could dominate.

In June 1972, a suit was brought in the U.S. District Court for Northern Florida by the American College of Nursing Home Administrators, the American Nursing Home Association, the State of Florida, the Florida Board of Nursing Home Examiners, the National Association of Boards of Examiners of Nursing Home Administrators, and the Florida Nursing Home Association against then-Secretary Elliot Richardson. The suit charged that HEW regulations encroached on the rights of the states to determine composition of the licensure boards. The Federal District Court ruled in favor of the Secretary, but the nursing home associations filed notice of appeal which was subsequently denied.

Just how far can the federal government go in regulating the nursing home industry? The issue is not totally decided, but the ability to control who or what receives federal funds gives real power to the federal government. If the federal government deems that the states fall short in fulfilling their obligations to care for their citizenry, and if society persists in its demands for a comprehensive long-term health care policy, the federal government will have to implement future policy decisions through its power of the purse.

THE PATIENT'S RIGHTS

There is a basic flaw in laws that give the nursing home patient rights to adequate medical care and other moral necessities. They assume that the individual has the ability to recognize shortcomings in care and treatment and, more significantly, that the patient is mentally or physically capable of acting to remedy the situation. Unfortunately, most nursing home patients are incapable of contesting their position. While most of them are there voluntarily, they are physically and financially powerless to get out.

Mary Mendelson writes,[6]

> People are in nursing homes because they have lost the power, physical or financial or both, to function independently, and it is because they are powerless that they are abused. Patients already have more rights, in the abstract, than they can use. No bars keep the patient in a home where he is abused; he is a prisoner of his own helplessness. He is in theory free to leave, but he cannot because he is sick or feeble, he is old, he has no money, and he has lost contact with the world outside. So he stays and accepts his abuse. No patient's organization, guarantee of legal rights, is going to change the realities of the nursing home patient's plight.

Even new laws that specifically address the rights of the nursing home patient can be of little help so long as no one has the desire or diligence to enforce them. Certainly nursing home patients are in no position to protect themselves from the abuses that a greedy system has spawned. If change is to come, it must come from other members of society, through passage and strict implementation of a genuine long-term health care policy.

CONCLUSIONS

Government control over the delivery of medical care in nursing homes has come as a result of the provision of public funds provided to pay for this care. Requirements governing the quality of care involve not only the delivery of care but also minimum standards for physical facilities and minimum levels of professional competency.

Nursing home patients are frequently unable to defend the rights provided them under the Medicare and Medicaid laws. The question, therefore, is how to preserve, protect, and defend these rights.

NOTES

1. National Center for Health Statistics (Washington, D.C.: U.S. Government Printing Office, 1978).
2. U.S. Senate, Subcommittee on Long–Term Care of the Special Senate Committee on Aging, "Nursing Home Care in the United States," 1965.
3. U.S. Senate Subcommittee on Long-Term Care of the Special Senate Committee on Aging, "Nursing Home Care in the United States: Failure in Public Policy," November 1974.
4. "Nursing Home Care in the United States," 1965.
5. M. A. Mendelson, *Tender Loving Greed* (New York: Alfred A. Knopf, 1974) p. xii.
6. Ibid., p. 240.

Chapter 14

Reorganizing the Nursing Home Industry: A Proposal*

In this chapter authors David Shulman and Ruth Galanter argue for a restructuring of the ownership of the physical facilities that house nursing homes. It is their thesis that once capital facilities are out of the hands of the nursing home operator, resources currently devoted to capital would be available for the provision of high quality patient care.

One of the main reasons behind the growth of private sector nursing homes, apart from the Medicare and Medicaid laws, is the way in which the capital facilities required for nursing homes can be used as tax shelters. The authors propose eliminating these tax shelters by establishing government agencies whose main function is to own the capital facilities. However, Shulman and Galanter suggest that the management and operation of the nursing homes remain in private hands to ensure that management remains competitive and cost-conscious, with built-in incentives for providing quality care.

David Shulman, Ph.D., is at the Graduate School of Administration, University of California at Riverside. Ruth Galanter, M.C.P., is with the National Health Law Program, Los Angeles, California.

OVERVIEW

This is a proposal to restructure the nursing home industry so that market forces will reinforce public policy objectives instead of impeding them, as they do at present. We propose a reorganization of the industry with capital facilities owned by government, rather than the private sector, but with management conducted through a system of competitive contracts with the private sector. This is not itself a solution to the problems of the nursing home care currently

* This chapter originally appeared as an article by David Shulman and Ruth Galanter, *Millbank Memorial Fund Quarterly (MMFQ) Health and Society* (Spring 1976): 129–43. It is reprinted with permission.

available, but it is prerequisite to solution; government ownership of capital facilities would transfer nursing home operators' financial incentives away from real estate investment and into patient care. At present, services already given must be reimbursed, regardless of the quality of those services or of pending action against the facility or operator. Consequently, abuses continue, and continue unpunished, long after they are discovered. The type of management contract we propose would require successful performance of the contract specifications in order to collect reimbursement and is thus an important handle for enforcing standards. This proposal should not be interpreted as a justification of nursing homes instead of alternative forms of care or as an argument that nursing homes can ever be truly satisfactory health care institutions.

The nursing home industry is a disaster, well documented by innumerable investigations and reports (U.S. Senate . . . , 1975; U.S. Department of Health, Education and Welfare, 1975).[1] Demands for reform, reasonably enough, have accompanied the recent disclosures of abuse, inadequacy, and cheating, and proposals for reform are legion. With a few exceptions (such as a "bill of rights" for nursing home patients), the reform proposals rely heavily on increased governmental supervision, regulation, and funds: more training programs for nursing home workers, more subsidies for building, more inspections, more elaborate record-keeping requirements.[2] Even assuming passage and adequate funding of these reforms, past experience in the nursing home industry and in other regulated industries suggests that this route alone is unreliable and definitely not cost-effective.

Government created, supports, and is ultimately responsible for the maintenance of the nursing home industry. Between 1960 (prior to Medicare and Medicaid) and 1974, nursing home care expenditures grew approximately 1400 percent (U.S. Senate . . . , 1975: I, 21). As of 1973, the country had 16,000 nursing homes with a total of 1,200,000 beds, generating $3.9 billion of revenue (Standard and Poor's Industry Surveys, 1974). In 1974, revenue had increased to $4.3 billion, and by 1975 revenue is estimated to hit $4.7 billion (Standard and Poor's Industry Surveys, 1975). If homes offering personal care (without nursing) and domiciliary care are included, the 1974 total is 22,000 (U.S. Department of Health, Education and Welfare, Public Health Service, 1974).

Three-quarters of the private nursing homes are operated on a for-profit basis (Standard and Poor's Industry Surveys, 1975). Although there remain a number of family-owned and managed nursing homes, most of the nursing home industry (measured in volume) is organized with the same split between ownership and management as the rest of American business. Nursing home operators can be expected to conduct themselves as "rational businesspeople." Failure to do so would lead to a foreclosure by the mortgage holder with a resulting loss of the facility. Or, at an earlier stage, a manager's failure to behave as a "rational businessperson" would lead to the owner's getting a new manager.

Nursing homes derive their basic authority to exist from state licensing requirements, administered by an agency of or delegated by state government. To be eligible for reimbursement under Medicare and/or Medicaid, nursing homes must be certified, by government, in a process separate from their regular licensing. The federal government has promulgated standards the homes must meet in order to be certified (Code of Federal Regulations [CFR], 1972; 1973); although the standards leave a lot to be desired, they are all the "law" there is.

Although the care is provided by private institutions, two-thirds of the industry's revenue comes from government, through Medicare, Medicaid, and other programs (Standard and Poor's Industry Surveys, 1975). Moreover, under the current fiscal structure, nursing home investors receive multiple subsidy: the reimbursement formulas include a percentage return on invested capital,[3] and the sheltering of income from taxation by investment in real estate means that the government foregoes taxes it would otherwise collect.[4] Both these forms of government subsidy provide government-funded income to entities which may have no interest or competence in nursing home care and no responsibility for nursing home care.

In some places, state government subsidizes construction of nursing homes and/or non-profit hospitals through medical care facilities finance agencies which provide up to 100 percent financing.[5]

Through inspection procedures, government is also ultimately responsible for maintenance of the facilities. Inspection for compliance with and enforcement of state and local building, fire, and other safety codes is usually done by state or local health departments, fire departments, building departments, or several of these agencies. When any of the responsible agencies conducts an inspection or review and finds a violation, it must follow specified procedures to induce change. All of these procedures take time, and the process can be turned off at any of the stages.[6] The entire process is easily abused through bribery or through the more subtle pressures that typically dilute the effectiveness of regulation (constant contact of regulators with regulatees and very little contact with those on whose behalf the regulators theoretically operate). But the problem is not only with individual inspectors; regulatory agencies frequently have official or unofficial policies in favor of negotiation rather than prosecution, and the resulting "political climate" makes termination of licensure or certification very difficult. In addition, current reimbursement structures preclude refusing to pay for services rendered during the decertification process.[7]

Enforcement of the applicable laws and standards by the public agencies responsible depends to a large extent on the level of staffing of those agencies, policy decisions with respect to techniques of enforcement, zeal in pursuing violators, and the prosecutors' and courts' diligence in following through on the agencies' complaints. In short, this process is time-consuming, expensive (staff time), unreliable (easily abused), and ineffective (U.S. Senate . . . , 1975).[8]

Private efforts to enforce even those standards which exist are still more limited. Employees are usually unorganized, ruling out collective action. Individual employees are extremely vulnerable to retaliation and usually badly need the jobs.[9] Patients and their families are usually desperately in need of help by the time they encounter the nursing home and therefore in no condition to assert themselves. Frequently they have no idea where to turn with a complaint. They also fear, with ample justification, retaliation against the patient (U.S. Senate . . . , 1975). Under some conditions, the patient or family may attempt a lawsuit for medical malpractice. Malpractice litigation is an extremely difficult process, however, and few people have real access to it even if they are willing to put up with the problems.[10] When the patient is elderly (as nearly 80 percent of nursing home patients are [U.S. Department of Health, Education and Welfare, 1975]), malpractice litigation is particularly difficult because the potential dollar amount of recovery is based in part on the potential earnings of which the malpractice victim was deprived by the act of malpractice. In short, for most nursing home patients, this enforcement route is effectively nonexistent.

Under the current structure of the nursing home industry, the normal forces of the marketplace create incentives which impede the achievement of government's stated policy objectives. They do this by forcing resources into the area of fixed costs (capital facilities) rather than variable costs (such as labor and food). In nursing homes, to a greater degree than in some other health care settings, the most important determinants of the quality of care are items of variable cost: the size of the labor force, the level of capability of the labor force (trained workers are more expensive than untrained ones), adequacy of diet, etc.[11] When these variable cost items are underfunded, patient care suffers. To understand the nature and functioning of these incentives, we have to move from the broad picture of the industry to a financial model of a typical nursing home bed.

FINANCIAL MODEL OF A TYPICAL NURSING HOME BED

The nursing home industry is capital-intensive; that is, the industry generates lower annual revenues than the capital required to generate those revenues. Much of the capital intensity is *not* due to investment in active capital equipment, but rather to investment in real estate.[12] In many ways, a nursing home is analogous to an investment in an apartment building or hotel. The financial model for a typical nursing home bed (see tables below) demonstrates that the Medicare/Medicaid reimbursements serve to validate the *real estate* value of a nursing home.

Table 14-1 Investment (Typical Nursing Home Bed)

1. Land	$ 500
2. Building	7,500
3. Total investment	$8,000

The model assumes that the nursing home bed is owned and operated on a for-profit basis, since three-fourths of all U.S. nursing home beds are so owned and operated. Although this model is incomplete to the extent that there are non-profit operators in the field, it does include those nursing homes owned by individual operators, by tax shelter syndicates, and by corporate chains.

The financial model is based on a composite taken from the Securities and Exchange Commission Forms 10K for National Health Enterprises, Charter Medical Corp., and Beverly Enterprises. These three publicly held companies control approximately 18,000 nursing home beds. Because the data were taken from forms for 1972 and 1973, investment and revenues are understated in terms of today's costs.

Table 14-1 shows the investment required per bed; and Table 14-2 shows how that typical bed is financed.

This typical nursing home bed generates net revenues of $16 per day, after an allowance-for-vacancy factor of approximately 8 percent (Standard and Poor's Industry Surveys, 1975).

Table 14-3 shows the annual income statement for the typical bed.

At first glance, Table 14-3 appears to show that the nursing home bed is only marginally profitable. A 4.1 percent profit margin, derived from pre-tax income (line 8) divided by net revenues (line 1), is lower than the profit margin in most capital-intensive industries. The 12 percent return on owner's equity can be considered a "normal" return in these days of high interest rates and is

Table 14-2 Financing (Typical Nursing Home Bed)

1. 9½%, 30-year first mortgage	$5,600[a]
2. 12% 20-year second mortgage	1,400
3. Total debt	7,000
4. Owner's equity	1,000
5. Total investment	$8,000

[a] 70% of total investment.

Table 14-3 Annual Income Statement (Typical Nursing Home Bed)

1. Net revenues @ $16/day	$5,840
2. Less: operating expenses	4,678
3. Net operating expenses	1,162
Capital Costs	
4. Depreciation (3% of building)	225[a]
5. Interest on first mortgage	530[b]
6. Interest on second mortgage	167[b]
7. Total capital costs	922
8. Pre-tax income (net operating income minus total capital costs)	240
9. Less: income taxes (approximately 50%)	120
10. Net income	$120[c]

[a] Assumes 33⅓ years useful life of building (Table 14-1, Line 2).
[b] First year's interest; thereafter it is lower.
[c] Assumes a 12% return on equity equal to one and one-half times the U.S. Treasury long-term bond interest rate as prescribed by Medicare.

consistent with Medicare reimbursement rates. If, as the table appears to show, return on investment was "normal" and in line with those in other industries competing for the investor's money, we would not be able to explain the rapid growth in the private nursing home industry. However, the income statement shows only part of the picture. For a more realistic understanding, we need in addition to examine a cash-flow statement, depicting the amount of cash the nursing home bed is generating. Real estate attracts a sizable number of investors; one of the main attractions of real estate as an investment is that it produces tax-sheltered cash flow, which can be used for other investments. Cash flow is the key factor in the evaluation of most real estate.

Table 14-4 shows the cash-flow statement of our typical nursing home bed.

In comparing the income statement with the cash-flow statement, the most important numbers are the ones which appear in only one table. The income statement, which lists income and expenses for tax purposes, includes depreciation (Table 14-3, line 4). Depreciation is a deductible expense for tax purposes and is based on historical cost. The higher the cost, the higher the depreciation deduction.[13] The cash-flow statement does not include depreciation because depreciation does not require cash outlay. Depreciation is only a bookkeeping deduction for allocating the building costs of Table 14-1. On the other hand, the cash-flow statement includes (but the income statement does not) an amount for repayment of the principal as well as the interest on the mortgage. Interest on the mortgage is deductible for tax purposes, but repayment of principal is not.

Table 14-4 Annual Cash Flow Statement (Typical Nursing Home Bed)

1. Net operating income (Table 14-3, line 3)		$1,162
Less: Cash Costs		
2. Interest on mortgages (Table 14-3, lines 5 and 6)	$697	
3. Principal amortization	53[a]	
4. Total mortgage payments	750	
5. Income taxes (Table 14-3, line 9)	120	
6. Total cash costs		870
7. Net cash flow (after tax)		$ 292
8. Percentage of owner's equity (Table 14-4, line 7, divided by Table 14-2, line 4)		29.2%

[a] First-year amortization; higher for later years.

(Repayment of principal is considered a capital transaction, which is neither income nor expense.) Thus, repayment of principal does not appear in the income statement as an expense, but it does appear in the cash-flow statement because it requires the outlay of cash.

As long as the depreciation is larger than the amortization of principal, the nursing home is generating cash flow in excess of net income. Cash flow can thus be positive while net income is negative.

Table 14-4 shows that our typical nursing home bed generates cash at the rate of 29 cents per dollar of investment. This is considered a very high return in both real estate and non-real-estate circles. This high return accounts for the large amount of capital attracted to the industry and thus for the industry's growth.

The cash generated is now available for whatever the owner may choose to do with it; investment in additional beds, distribution to the owners, or investment in other types of property. Beverly Enterprises, for instance, used its cash flow to invest in second-home developments in northern California.

IMPLICATIONS

The financial model demonstrates that the factor that attracts capital into the nursing home-business is not net income but net cash flow. Net cash flow is based in large measure on the depreciation deductions which are bookkeeping matters unrelated to a reduction in economic value, not real cash outlays. Thus, in order to increase net cash flow, the nursing home entrepreneur wants the highest possible depreciable basis per dollar of owner's equity.

Once the depreciable basis is in place, the entrepreneur seeks to maintain a net operating income sufficient to cover his or her mortgage payments. This process validates the market value of the nursing home real estate by assuring a tax-sheltered cash flow to the owner.

There are only two ways to accomplish this: maximize income and/or minimize expenses. To maximize income, the operator will try to maintain high rates of occupancy and to promote increases in the reimbursement rates under Medicare and Medicaid. To reduce expenses, the operator will try to cut those costs which are flexible enough to cut, specifically operating costs.[14] This can be done by using low-cost labor, by providing only a minimal diet, and by skimping on all sorts of services including maintenance. In the current economic climate, when state legislatures are especially reluctant to spend additional funds, the only practical method is to reduce operating expenses to the barest minimum. (The same economic climate that makes legislatures reluctant to raise reimbursement rates also makes them reluctant to allocate additional funds to inspection of nursing homes and processing of compliants and violations.)

Although some reductions in operating expenses may well be justified economies, evidence presented to the various investigations of nursing home care suggests that this tendency to reduce operating expenses has very serious health care costs and human consequences. In order to retain control of the nursing home, the operator must maintain a net operating income sufficient to cover the mortgage payments. This is true for all real estate. However, because of the unique Medicaid payment process for nursing homes which generally makes it difficult to increase prices (rent) in the short run, the operator has no choice but to minimize operating expenses (refer to footnote 4). It is in the minimizing of operating expenses that the quality of care is reduced. This does not necessarily make the operator a "villain"; the operator is literally forced into this course of action by the economics of the industry as it is presently structured.

From this examination, it is clear that real estate, not patient care, is the name of the game. We propose to change the game, to permit focus of both the funds and the efforts on the stated policy objectives, namely high-quality nursing home care of patients.

OUR PROPOSAL

Capital facilities, specifically real estate, would be owned by government. Management, however, would be carried out by the private sector through a competitive process designed to improve the quality of management and to encourage performance monitoring by private individuals and groups as well as government agencies.

Once capital facilities (and thus also the real estate aspects of nursing home operation) are out of the hands of the operator, the incentives that currently impede provision of high quality care by diverting resources to capital are also removed. In addition, the taxes presently avoided by those investing in nursing home real estate as a tax shelter can also be collected.[15]

Because government has a strong tendency to devitalize any system it runs for any length of time, and because government management prevents competition and its attendant benefits, we stop at public *ownership*. (Considering the extent of government participation in the industry at present, this is actually quite a small step.)

For management, we propose a system of contracts with private management corporation (either profit-making or non-profit). This is similar to non-profit hospitals (such as those owned by religious orders) contracting with private, profit-making management firms for operation of their hospitals. In designing this aspect of the system, the most critical considerations are the contract specifications, the methods of achieving full public exposure of everything that happens during the operation of the system, and the creation of genuine competition.

Contracts would have minimum performance specifications, with bonuses for proven past successes or for arguably beneficial innovations. Contracts would also have specified limited duration, so that at intervals the performance of the contractor could be officially and publicly reviewed and the contract again put up for competitive bid. The previous holder of the contract could of course compete for the upcoming contract, along with anyone else meeting certain limited qualifications.

Since capital assets would no longer be required of the private contractor, entry into the business would be relatively easy in terms of capital requirements. This would allow many management groups to enter the bidding process, assuring a high degree of competition. The current system requires a substantial real estate investment prior to licensing.

The contract-award process, with its required new bidding at each interval, would serve as a brake on unforeseen abuses. This system also has the distinct advantage that it permits competing away potential monopoly profits earned by the management company.[16] If "excess" profits are earned, they would presumably be competed away at the next contract award.

The differences between the proposed and the existing system can be seen by returning to Table 14-3. In the proposed system, we are concerned only with lines 1 to 3. Capital costs are no longer relevant to the operator and thus, in order to fulfill the contractual obligations to provide care, the operator is concerned only with line 2 (operating expenses). This is, in fact, the only item which is involved in the contract. As long as the operator fulfills its contractual obligations, the state should be satisfied.

Like any owner of a service establishment, government would remain responsible for the quality of management provided in its establishments even though it did not itself carry out the management function. Under the proposed system, however, fulfillment of this responsibility would be greatly simplified. The ultimate test of management effectiveness is the quality of care provided to the nursing home patient. Government would have three major ways to ensure the quality of care. To begin with, government would draw up the contract specifications, presumably using the advice of people who know something about what makes high-quality care. Second, the competitive bidding process for the award of contracts would permit replacing an inadequate manager with a better one. There would no longer be a need for government to prove malice or neglect; the contract would simply end at the specified time with no promises of renewal. Previous holders of management contracts would not have vested rights in those contracts. Since the contractors would have no investment in the facility, changeover to a new contractor would be simple. Inadequate operations would exist, at most, only for the length of the contract. With a well-designed process for review of performance with widespread dissemination of information about what is going on, and for effective public participation, market forces can be used to assist government in selecting those managers who provide high-quality care. Instead of relying only on patients and inspectors for word of contract violations, government would now also have available the resources of competitors for the contract. Firms anxious to succeed in the nursing home management business would have strong financial incentives to report their competitors' failings through the public-review/contract-award process. Thus, the periodic review process could serve as a market test of the efficiency and quality of the care provided.

Finally, the legal relationship between nursing homes and the government would be greatly simplified. Instead of relying on withdrawal of Medicare/Medicaid reimbursements, and in some cases on criminal sanctions, the government would now be in a position to enforce its rights through the civil courts under contract law. This legal process is a great deal easier to implement than the old one, hence the risk to the nursing home operator of violating the contract is substantially greater than before. Failure to fulfill the contract as specified is a breach of contract and subject to civil penalties. More immediately, withholding of the final installment of payment is entirely proper if the contract was not fulfilled.

This system is quite similar to the franchise bidding system outlined by Demsetz (1968) in his proposal for the utility industry. Although there are substantial differences between the nursing home industry and the utility industry, there are strong similarities: a long history of government regulation, essentialness of the service, and the relatively high proportion of total assets invested in capital facilities. Demsetz's system requires two explicit assumptions: (1) the inputs required to enter production must be available to many potential bidders at prices determined in open markets, and (2) the cost of collusion by bidding rivals must be prohibitively high.

Our proposal for nursing homes would, we believe, meet those conditions, first, by the elimination of substantial capital requirements as an entry barrier, and second, by the large number of facilities within a given market area. Also the periodic-review process, coupled with the ease of entry, would tend to mitigate against collusion by bidders. In addition, monopolistic control on the capacity of the industry would be exercised by government, thus preventing over-bedding in some areas and underbedding in others, greatly simplifying the organization of health planning and presumably reducing overall system-wide vacancies.

Under this structure, we are out of the real estate net-cash-flow arena. With that change, the incentives which currently impede provision of high-quality care by diverting resources to capital are also removed. With these out of the way, it is now possible for both government and the private sector to address the stated public policy objective of high-quality patient care. If, as a nation, we are still unable to solve the major problems which currently plague nursing home patients, we will have to examine whether the stated public policy objectives are in fact the real public policy objectives.

NOTES

1. See also *New York Times* (1975: 1804-1807). Of the various references listed there, see especially the October 7-10 four-part investigative series and stories beginning October 17 on the New York State Temporary Committee on Living Costs.

2. Senator Moss, Representatives Abzug and Koch, and others have already introduced in Congress close to 50 bills dealing with nursing home reform. Some types of reforms have been instituted. In New York, for instance, the state is now required to perform quality assessment as part of its regular review.

3. Medicare reimburses according to a cost formula which includes depreciation, interest on debt, and a return on owner's equity of one and one-half times the long-term U.S. Treasury bond interest rate as allowable costs. Medicaid reimburses on a per day capitation payment basis, with the amount of the payment determined by the state government.

4. Real estate investment is especially attractive to people in high tax brackets, and the marketing of such investment opportunities is directed to such people. For an example of how nursing homes fit in, see Needham (1969).

5. The New York State Medical Care Facilities Finance Agency grants 90-100 percent financing to non-profit nursing homes. (With 100 percent financing, there is no owner's equity involved.) In April 1975, that agency sold $62 million in revenue bonds whose proceeds were allocated to the construction of non-profit hospitals and nursing homes. A total of $14.7 million was allocated for nursing homes (New York State Medical Care Facilities Finance Agency,

Hospital and Home Project Bonds, 1975 Series A, Prospectus, April 23, 1975). As a result of New York's financial troubles, this agency has been unable to sell additional bonds. However, the Illinois Health Facilities Authority, the Connecticut Health and Educational Facilities Authority, and the Philadelphia Hospitals Authority successfully sold bonds in 1975.

6. Inspection for compliance with and enforcement of these types of standards is generally done by the state or local health departments. In addition, there are standards which may be within the purview of the local building department or the local fire department. When any of the responsible agencies conducts an inspection or review and finds a violation, it must follow specified procedures to induce change. If all proceeds normally, however, there will usually be a notice provision specifying a time period for correcting the deficiency. Then there must be a reinspection. There may be "second notice" procedures. Finally, though, there is the power of prosecution. However, prosecutors are generally not from the same agencies as the inspectors. Inspectors merely file complaints with prosecutors. Prosecutors have other things to think about besides nursing homes, and they are not always anxious to prosecute—particularly when both they and the courts view the issues as essentially civil rather than criminal. Even if they do prosecute, the case may take months to come to resolution and the fine may be quite minimal. Even when the process works completely on schedule, throughout the court proceedings the violation may remain uncorrected.

7. Under CFR 20 405.604, 615 all services prior to decertification are reimbursed by Medicare and Medicaid (Code of Federal Regulations [CFR], 1972). In addition, payments are made for another 30 days after an intent to decertify is announced.

8. California has instituted a tougher system, but there has not yet been enough experience to evaluate the results.

9. For an example of instructions to nursing home operators for dealing with labor, see Needham (1969: 137–200).

10. Only those cases with high potential recovery reach litigation, because the lawyer's fee is determined by the amount of recovery, and lawyers do not typically undertake the extensive preparation necessary for successful litigation unless the fee will make it worthwhile.

11. In hospitals, for instance, complex and expensive equipment (capital) may be at least equally important in determining the quality of care available.

12. In contrast, the utility industry (also capital-intensive) requires proportionately heavy investments in production equipment.

13. This tax-accounting notion can lead to the repeated sale of nursing homes at ever higher prices with Medicare reimbursing at ever higher rates. As long as Medicare/Medicaid reimbursements are sufficient to cover this "higher" depreciation, the higher sale price of the nursing home is validated.

14. Capital costs are fixed and thus cannot be reduced.

15. Although the property taxes now paid by proprietary homes would no longer be collected, an in lieu fee could be required. This would offset property tax revenue, but the income previously sheltered in the real estate investment would not be subject to income tax.

16. This contrasts with California's prepaid health plan (PHP) contracting in several important ways. PHP contractors must either own or contract for substantial capital facilities: nursing home contractors will own none. PHP contractors generally negotiate their contracts with the state on an exclusive, non-competitive basis. Nursing home contractors would compete. In practice, the complete PHP contract file is not generally available to the public. The nursing home bids would become public as soon as the bidding period closed, and the entire file would be public.

REFERENCES

Code of Federal Regulations (CFR), *Employees Benefits*, Volume 20 (Washington, D.C.: U.S. Government Printing Office, 1972).

Public Welfare, Volume 45 (Washington, D.C.: U.S. Government Code of Federal Regulations (CFR), Printing Office, 1973).

Demsetz, Harold, "Why regulate utilities?" *Journal of Law and Economics* 11 (April 1968): 55-65.

Needham, Roger A. (ed.), *Nursing Homes: Legal and Business Problems* (New York: Practicing Law Institute, 1969).

New York Times Index 1974, Volume II (New York: New York Times, 1975).

Standard and Poor's, *Health Care*. H 23 (New York: Standard and Poor's, 1974).

Standard and Poor's, *Health Care*. H 23, 24 (New York: Standard and Poor's, 1975).

U.S. Department of Health, Education and Welfare, *Long Term Care Facility Improvement Study* (July) (Washington, D.C.: U.S. Government Printing Office, 1975).

U.S. Department of Health, Education and Welfare, Public Health Service, *Health Resource Statistics* (Rockville, Maryland: U.S. Department of Health, Education and Welfare, Public Health Service, Health Resources Administration, National Center for Health Statistics, 1974).

U.S. Senate, Special Committee on Aging, Subcommittee on Long Term Care, *Nursing Home Care in the United States: Failure in Public Policy. Introductory Report and Supporting Papers.* (Washington, D.C.: U.S. Government Printing Office, 1975).

Chapter 15

A National Health Policy for the Aged

T his chapter examines how a health policy for the elderly can be developed. The elderly are heavy consumers of health care, and public funds finance most of this care. How can existing agencies (such as the Health Systems Agencies) and existing institutions (such as nursing homes) be utilized in implementing a national health policy for the aged?

Health care for the elderly, like related programs of social services and income maintenance, are rather fragmented. Presently health care is expensive at all levels, is not always of good quality, and frequently is delivered inappropriately. With the large amounts of public funds being spent on the aged, and numerous government and private entities participating in these programs, it is not surprising that the current system is not cost-effective. Neither does it represent a rational or comprehensive approach to providing health services for the nation's elderly. Government bureaucracies, conflicting legislation, and a myriad of regulations and local-state-federal power struggles have stymied any progress in formulating and discussing the issues surrounding social policy for the elderly. For example, the following "remedies" have been suggested (and some implemented) to ameliorate the problem of providing institutional care for the elderly:[1]

- reimbursing nursing homes at cost and applying what are regarded as stringent regulations

- an experiment with extended care to determine and utilize a system of equitable cost reimbursement together with a system for utilization review in relation to secondary care institutions

- relating rates of reimbursement for institutional care to the amount of care the patient required. These systems have been characterized as "point-count systems" with so many points for incontinence, for immobility, for inability to dress, feed oneself, etc.

- training and education programs in Pennsylvania and California in conjunction with some form of the above remedies
- methods intended to improve competitioh to assure high quality care at reasonable cost. These have included FHA mortgage and Hill-Burton grants to relieve the shortage of skilled nursing home beds
- appointment of a special assistant to the Secretary of HEW for nursing home affairs; administrative attempts through Medicaid regulation enforcement to upgrade nursing homes as part of federal efforts; the training of state inspectors and nursing home administrators with federal funds.

Since the time these remedies were suggested, there have been considerable improvements in regulations for quality and cost control. However, the problems of health care for the elderly extend well beyond the realm of the nursing home patient. Home health care, day health care, and routine ambulatory care also need to be addressed.

A NATIONAL HEALTH POLICY FOR THE ELDERLY

A national health policy for the elderly must consider the input as well as the needs of state and local governments. It is one task to develop a national policy; it is a totally different task to implement that policy.

One vehicle to use for state-by-state and area-by-area implementation is the Health Systems Agency (HSA) or its successor. The word "successor" reminds one that regional health planning has evolved over time. It appears that the current Health Systems Agency, brought into being by P.L. 93-641 during the mid-1970s, is only one step in the evolutionary process. It can be said that regional health planning began with the Hill-Burton Act, since Hill-Burton funds for hospital construction also involved the commitment of considerable local and state funds. In the mid-1960s the Regional Medical Programs and the Comprehensive Health Planning Agencies (CHPA) were brought into being through federal legislation. The CHPA was most closely related to the present Health System Agency. In fact, the CHPA of the Sixties was transformed into the HSA of the Seventies. Therefore, it seems likely that a successor to the HSA will evolve during the mid-1980s.

The duties of the local Health Systems Agency are manyfold but can be summarized by the following ongoing activities:

- develop a Regional Health Systems Plan
- develop an Annual Implementation Plan
- review all Capital Expenditure Programs
- provide technical assistance for grant proposals
- review all grant and loan requests.

At first glance it may appear that the local Health Systems Agency has considerable power. In fact, the power is relatively limited, and nonauthorization of grants, loans, or capital projects can be overturned by federal or state political intervention.

According to Waters and Tierney[2] state and local health systems planning has not been successful in the United States because of the lack of financial incentives. It is their contention that an economic stimulus is mandatory to ensure decentralized health systems planning. By allocating a finite health budget to the states and allowing the states to decide—within certain boundaries and norms—how to allocate those budgets, serious health planning at the state and local level will be possible. If these steps are not taken, local decision makers will not take health planning very seriously. Waters and Tierney conclude by stating that successful health planning is based on enlightened self-interest. As long as the states are penalized financially by the federal government for rational health planning, the states will continue to *conduct planning games* while pursuing *more pragmatic decision rules* at the same time. Planning games are responses to federal regulations and bureaucratic requirements that will ensure that the maximum amount of federal assistance is obtained.

How do these recommendations affect state or regional planning for health care for the elderly? If the Waters and Tierney suggestions were adopted, and assuming that the "boundaries and norms" included consideration of health care needs unique to the elderly, there should be some improvements in the delivery of health care to the elderly. Unique needs such as day health care, home health care, and institutional care could become beneficiaries of a state or regional health plan.

At present, however, under the conditions of P.L. 93-641, the benefits to be derived from regional health planning may be somewhat limited. Areawide health planning by the HSA intends to integrate the input of various interest groups at the community level. P.L. 93-641 was passed by Congress in order to provide communities with the incentive to initiate a systemized plan for health care delivery. This law, and the trend it represents, will undoubtedly affect the type and method of care the elderly receive. P.L. 93-641 provides opportunities for the development of efficient health care delivery systems and the elimination of unnecessary duplication. The number of institutional alternatives for providing care may be reduced if regional planning studies determine they are redundant.

In enacting the provisions of P.L. 93-641, Congress found that a massive infusion of federal funds into the existing health care system has only contributed to the inflationary spiral in health care and failed to produce an adequate supply or distribution of health resources. In recognition of the magnitude of these problems and the importance of a quick solution, P.L. 93-641 intends to be the driving force that facilitates the development of recommendations for a national health planning policy. As part of the act, areawide and statewide planning for health services, manpower, and facilities will be augmented. The functions of the HSA and the State Health Planning and Development Agency include cost-containment provisions for providing health services and the preventing unnecessary duplication of health resources. Such functions improve patient care services for the elderly and are consistent with the intent of provider reimbursement policy under the Medicare program.

OBSTACLES TO IMPLEMENTING NATIONAL HEALTH POLICY

The present system that delivers health care to the elderly leaves much to be desired. Institutionalization in nursing homes is common for the approximately 5 percent of elderly who need constant personal care. The alternatives to institutionalization (such as home health care, day health care, and organized ambulatory care) are largely experimental at present.

The changes that have taken place since the Health System Agency arrived in the mid-1970s can at best be referred to as *incrementalism*. Incrementalism is a term made prominent by Lindblom.[3] It is a more modern and democratic version of Edmund Burke's idea that the best of all possible worlds is the one that is now. In terms of health care for the elderly, it means that legislators will argue with one another until they reach a resulting compromise that adds just a "bit" more to the elderly's pie. The quality of that "bit," or broader questions of whether and what the elderly need in terms of health care, is not always considered.

To illustrate this point, consider the issue of institutionalized versus noninstitutionalized care for the elderly. While there is still some dispute over costs, the weight of evidence favors noninstitutionalized care on a per person basis. Others argue that care would have to be extended to include such services as day care and home care, and as a result the pool of prospective claimants would dramatically expand. This would lead to a tremendous increase in total expenditures for health care. But if society, in fact, feels a social responsibility to its aged population, then it must translate that concern into action through broader coverage. In terms of implementation, that coverage is best represented by a national program to expand day care and home care. Costs could still be contained through rigorous screening and through incentives that encourage families to continue care of elderly relatives.

As long as health care is delivered and fragmented not only by various agencies but by similar agencies at various levels of government, well-rounded, quality care cannot be delivered and costs cannot be contained.

Financial incentives pose yet another obstacle to the development of a more desirable system. Public reimbursement methods follow three models:

1. cost-related payment mechanisms such as found in Medicare
2. flat rate payment mechanisms such as those used in Pennsylvania and Texas Medicaid
3. point count payment mechanisms that assess the needs of patients and pay accordingly, such as found in Illinois Medicaid.

In none of the three models is it to the advantage of a nursing home to discharge a patient at the earliest possible moment, to involve a patient in an appropriate day care or home care program, or to suggest or arrange for other noninstitutional services. Very few communities have a patient assessment and placement system that links admission and alternative treatment processes with reimbursement. Also, the promulgation of standards and regulations that are contingent upon payment have often built inflexibility into the system.

At a lower echelon, there is a whole new set of obstacles. It has been said that the objectives for long-term nursing home care are not clear. Hospital and primary care involve providing a "cure," but long-term care should have rehabilitation, physical restoration (short of return to self-care), life and activity maintenance, or support outside of a nursing home as objectives of treatment. But chronic nature of many of the elderly person's ailments means that objectives fluctuate with the needs of the patient. There is no single "cure" objective as with most acute illnesses.

Custom and experience usually determines what goals health professionals select as appropriate for long-term programs. In a hospital, for example, technological innovations are usually adopted quickly. This ability to respond quickly and correctly in hospitals enables a reasonable determination of such things as whether surgery is to be performed or what level of care is to be provided for certain types of illness.

In long-term care programs—whether they be day care, home care, or nursing home programs—there frequently is little understanding of the people who are served. Especially in the case of nursing home patients, there is a reluctance to participate in their care and frequently a sense of hopelessness and futility about investing energy and resources. There is also a lack of knowledge about the nature of many of their diseases and about their tolerance or susceptibility for surgery and rehabilitative techniques. Staff persons believe that most elderly patients are confused and without social utility. These attitudes and misconceptions are founded in the attitudes that society as a whole possesses. These beliefs have been, and will continue to be, a fundamental stumbling block in the development of the conventional wisdom necessary to cope with the problems of the aged.

THE NEED TO EVALUATE PROGRAMS OF TREATMENT ALTERNATIVES

There is yet another obstacle to the formation of a national health policy for the aged—a deficiency in basic knowledge. There is a general lack of information about what treatments are available for particular conditions and/or the value of any given treatment. Program evaluation procedures are, for the most part, nonexistent. Measurement that does occur is only a count of numbers served. What is required is unbiased appraisal of treatment alternatives in terms of their total value. This kind of evaluation will help answer that all-important question: Is it worth it? [4]

The development of these evaluation programs will require in-depth analysis of the elderly population. More needs to be known about those who require long-term care and those who have disabling conditions but are not actively seeking access to long-term care institutions. Similarly, more has to be known about the institutions themselves, their relationship to other long-term service systems, their operational incentives, and their manpower requirements. The establishment of these data bases will help overcome the barriers that stand in the way of developing a national health policy.

Tied to the evaluation issue is the important question of control. Who will determine the priorities? Who will implement them? What methods will be used? A wholistic approach calls for priorities to be set nationally, while implementation must be a function performed jointly by federal and state agencies and state and local agencies. A recent study at the University of Pennsylvania[5] highlighted the following issues:

> What implications do alternative control structures have on the nature of political and professional accountability regarding programs for the elderly? To what extent does an increased role for citizens' advisory boards translate into client representation and improved services as opposed to a provider or administrator-dominated "rubber stamp?" To what degree might control structures be adjusted from one local area to another to reflect the needs and demonstrated service capabilities in different local settings? What effect do control structures have on the capabilities of agency directors to carry out the goal of effectively coordinating a variety of other programs and services? . . . Clearly the issue of local control and the role of local government in health and health related services for the elderly needs much greater attention across the nation as the multiple objectives of accessibility are pursued.

A DEMONSTRATION PROJECT

With the inadequacies of the present system in mind, a community-wide demonstration project was undertaken by the New York State Department of Social Services.[6] The project's objective was "to develop community-wide, population-based models for the organization, delivery, and financing of long-term care for the aged that would prove to be more cost-effective and of better quality than the existing system." It was hypothesized by those developing the project that inflexibility of incentives is the major problem confronting the development of a long-term public policy.

> The most basic problem appears to be inability of local communities to organize and manage the provision and payment for long-term care in the face of specific and restrictive requirements imposed by Federal and state statute and regulation. The aged and chronically ill reside in local communities, where they need and use locally available health care resources. But federal and state program requirements have abrogated any community decision-making process that might be more sensitive to the needs of its residents. Detailed standards and classifications of providers, establishment of rates of payments, restrictive benefit definitions, multiple administrative responsibility, all tend to make the community impotent in taking a flexible approach to long-term care geared to patient needs, health care resources and fiscal constraints.[7]

The project intended to overcome some of these constraints by waiving certain federal regulations. In this manner, the participating communities and organizations can select and manipulate the services delivery and reimbursement model that is most appropriate. In this project and others like it, one sees the development of models that select variables or combinations of variables from a continuum that ranges from nearly no change to a system that is radically different from the present organization, delivery, and financing of health care for the aged.

CONCLUSIONS

This chapter has analyzed the barriers that stand in the way of long-term care national health policy for the elderly. Programs designed with these obstacles in mind have a much greater chance of success.

On a higher level, policy makers must determine the broad goals and social values that are a necessary component of sound national policy. Policy must be comprehensive and wholistic and not be a result of political pressure. Of course, bureaucracies and various state and local agencies cannot be allowed to distort the goals of national policy through infighting and unnecessary competition.

One approach calls for the implementation of demonstration projects similar to the one conducted by the New York Department of Social Services. By trying different approaches to the delivery of long-term care, we can discover the methods that most closely approach the ideal. Perhaps community per capita reimbursement, direct and increasing payment with age, institutional prepayment plans, or complete and strict federal regulation will do the best job. An improved long-term care system for the elderly will come out of experimentation with some of these new ideas.

NOTES

1. S. J. Brody and E. Cohen, ''Broad Social Issues,'' in *A Social Work Guide for Long-Term Care Facilities*, edited by Elaine M. Brody, National Institute of Mental Health (Washington, D.C.: U.S. Government Printing Office, 1974), p. 206-207.

2. W. J. Waters, and J. T. Tierney, ''Health Planning and National Health Insurance,'' *Inquiry* 15 (September 1978): 207.

3. Charles Lindblom, *The Policy-Making Process* (Englewood Cliffs, N.J.: Prentice-Hall, 1968).

4. *Evaluative Research on Social Programs for the Elderly*, U.S. Department of Health, Education and Welfare, Administration on Aging (Washington, D.C.: U.S. Government Printing Office, 1977).

5. L. Gamm and F. Eisele, ''The Aged and Chronically Ill,'' in *Health Services* (edited by Arthur Levin) (New York: Political Science Academy, 1977), p. 181.

6. *A Demonstration of Community-Wide Alternative Long Term Care Models*, New York State Department of Social Services, Albany, 1975.

7. Ibid., p. 18.

Chapter 16

Vision, Hearing, and Dental Care

T he U.S. House of Representatives Subcommittee on Health and Long Term Care of the Select Committee on Aging has investigated the needs of the elderly in terms of hearing aids, eyeglasses, and dentures as well as the high cost of these medical appliances. In September 1976 it published a report titled "Medical Appliances and the Elderly: Unmet Needs and Excessive Costs for Eyeglasses, Hearing Aids, Dentures and Other Devices."[1]

It was found that the well-being of virtually all of the 22.4 million elderly (in 1975) is dependent on one or more medical appliances. But the subcommittee found that the elderly's needs are not entirely met for two reasons: (1) There is a lack of federal assistance to help the elderly obtain desperately needed devices. Many of the elderly cannot afford the devices, and public and private health benefit programs have provided only limited help in this area. (2) There is a lack of adequate safeguards to protect them from abuses in purchasing these health aids. Those elderly who can afford them or that forgo other needs to acquire these appliances frequently are victims of overpricing and delivery of unnecessary goods or services.

In the area of vision care, about 90 percent of the elderly require and own eyeglasses. However, over five million elderly are wearing eyeglasses that need correction. In cases where there is a conflict of interest (such as an optometrist who provides both the eye examination and the eyeglasses), there is a high incidence of unnecessary prescriptions. Overpricing was discovered in numerous surveys conducted in various parts of the country.

Not so many of the elderly have hearing problems as have vision problems. However, about 50 percent of the elderly have some hearing impairment, and about 8 percent have severe hearing problems. Conflicts of interest are also common in the hearing aid industry. Although it is recommended that the customer consult an otolaryngologist or an otologist (both physicians), frequently hearing aids are purchased without medical intervention. The hearing aid dealer frequently selects the hearing aid for the customer, possibly providing an unnecessary or inappropriate medical device. Overpricing is also a common problem in the hearing aid industry.

During the mid-1970s, over half of the people over age 65 had no natural teeth. Over 5 percent of those elderly without teeth had no dentures; many of those with dentures had problems with their dentures that needed correction. The cost of acquiring, replacing, or repairing dentures is considerable. The elderly on limited budgets would, therefore, forgo dental care rather than commit more than they can afford to take care of their needs.

In all of the above cases, little or no financial assistance is available from private or public health benefit programs. In some states Medicaid will cover some of the unmet needs, but only for those elderly eligible for Medicaid.

The information contained in this chapter summarizes the report by the House Subcommittee on Health and Long Term Care.

VISION CARE AND EYEGLASSES

Vision care, including the prescription and acquisition of eyeglasses, is probably the single need that virtually all elderly share. The magnitude of this need is demonstrated by the following conditions. Next to arthritis, chronic vision impairment is the most common ailment of the elderly. Vision deteriorates with age, and as a result there are more cases of eye problems among the aged than among any other segment of the population. About 25 percent of the elderly need new corrective lenses because their present eyeglasses do not help their sight and in some cases may actually impair it. Many other elderly persons need eyeglasses but currently do not have them.

Many of the eye problems the elderly have need early and constant attention so that blindness does not result. In particular, glaucoma and senile cataracts should be diagnosed early so that proper treatments can be prescribed to avoid severe and nonreversible vision impairment. The rate of blindness in those over 65 is over 12 percent; these blindness conditions frequently are caused by untreated glaucoma and cataract conditions.

Although about 12 percent of the elderly are legally blind, an additional 8 percent have chronic vision impairments. It is generally believed that many cases of vision impairment can be corrected but that the costs of vision care and eyeglasses inhibit the elderly from seeking such care. Medicare and private insurance generally do not provide coverage for eyeglasses and vision checkups. Only under Medicaid in some states is vision care and eyeglasses a covered benefit.

The cost of vision care to the elderly is inflated for two reasons: (1) prescription of the wrong lenses, and (2) excessive cost for eyeglasses. Extensive investigations by the New York Department of Consumer Affairs have revealed that optometrists frequently prescribe the wrong lenses or prescribe eyeglasses in cases where none are required. It was found that many of the wrong prescriptions were not intentional but were the result of poor or inadequate conditions in the optometrist's office. Poor lighting and improperly focused eye charts frequently contributed to this situation.

There is serious evidence that overpricing of eyeglasses is common and rampant. Price variations of 200 percent, and occasionally as high as 300 percent, are common. Price variations of this magnitude clearly cannot be justified on the basis of differences in costs or overhead. The only conclusion is that serious overpricing exists. Unsuspecting elderly clients often are the victims of this overpricing and usually do not discover they have been victimized until it is too late.

How, then, can the elderly avoid becoming victims of these practices? It appears that information dissemination is probably the best approach. If the elderly knew which optometrists were unqualified or tended to overprice, they could avoid them. The problem is who will gather the information and disseminate it? The logical agency is the local Office or Department of the Aging. Another possibility is the elderly themselves. Through senior citizen centers, the elderly could develop lists of vision care providers who are qualified and trustworthy. Without an organized system by which they can disseminate information the elderly will become victims of overpricing—and overpricing inhibits the elderly from searching out much needed vision care.

HEARING CARE AND HEARING AIDS

According to the Federal Council on the Aging and the American Speech and Hearing Association, over 50 percent of people age 65 and older suffer from impaired hearing. For 8 percent of those 65 and over, the impairment is serious enough that they are unable to hear words that are spoken at a normal voice level. The solution in these cases is a suitable hearing aid. Unfortunately, hearing aids are expensive and few health benefit programs cover the acquisition and fitting of a hearing aid. As a result, for those unable to afford the hearing aid, the only alternative is to forgo it.

Hearing impairment takes a variety of forms. The first is an inability to hear speech and other sounds loudly enough. This is referred to as a "loss in hearing sensitivity" or simply "hearing loss." A second form of hearing impairment is an inability to hear speech and other sounds clearly, even though the sounds are sufficiently loud. This is referred to as "speech discrimination." Not having a hearing aid when it definitely is required poses a number of problems, including feelings of isolation, loneliness, and degradation.

The likelihood of having a serious impairment rises sharply with increased age. Only about 2.6 percent of persons between 12 and 24 years of age have serious hearing problems; in the 45 to 64 age bracket, the percentage increases to 10 percent; in those 65 years of age and over, 17.3 percent have serious hearing impairments. According to the National Health Survey conducted in the mid-1970s, slightly over a million of those in this last group were using hearing aids.

Because of the high cost of hearing aids, the hearing aid delivery system has been the subject of numerous investigators. Such groups as the Retired Professional Action Group (RPAG)—a nonprofit consumer advisory group, and the Subcommittee on Consumer Interests of the Elderly—Senate Special Committee on Aging, launched or caused the launching of other investigations. In 1973 the RPAG published a report entitled "Paying through the Ear: A Report on Hearing Health Care Problems." The report of the hearings of the Senate Subcommittee was entitled "Hearing Aids and Older Americans." These two reports inspired a HEW investigation that resulted in a 1975 report entitled "Final Report to the Secretary on Hearing Aid Health Care." All of these investigations and reports concluded that there are serious abuses in the way hearing aids are sold, and these abuses demand correction.

Oversell was the most serious problem uncovered. Because it is in the interest of the hearing aid seller to make a sale, sales frequently are made to people who do not really need them. In a sense this is not a health care problem, but an economic or fraud problem. The Senate Subcommittee proposed requiring a medical examination before a hearing aid could be sold. Although this would provide some degree of protection, it would also increase the cost of acquiring a hearing aid. A compromise solution was reached whereby patients were permitted to waive the medical examination if there were no obvious and clear medical problems present.

There are also considerable questions about the competency of hearing aid dealers. Although there is an instructional course for hearing aid dealers, the course has been seriously criticized. The National Hearing Aid Society (NHAS) in the mid-1970s offered a home study course consisting of 20 lessons. However, the Veterans Administration, the American Council of Otolaryngology, and the American Speech and Hearing Association severely criticized this course as inadequate, too technical for most participants, and superficial.

There were also questions of pricing. Retail costs of hearing aids were found to be up to two and one-half times the wholesale costs. The National Hearing Aid Society has defended these high costs on the basis of the markups required to cover the costs of such services as audiological tests, fitting, counseling about hearing aid use, and post-delivery services.

What about economies of scale? Could the cost of hearing aids be reduced through larger delivery centers? At present the hearing aid delivery system at the retail level is largely a "cottage industry." Entry of nonprofit corporations or large scale national franchising could very well lower costs considerably. But there is little indication at present that this is about to take place.

DENTAL CARE AND DENTURES

As recently as the mid-1970s, half of the U.S. population over 65 was edentulous (without any natural teeth). Although a majority of these people had dentures, the cost of acquiring dentures can be a considerable economic barrier to the older person on a limited budget. There are very few health benefit programs that cover dental care, and in virtually all cases the individuals are personally responsible for the acquisition costs.

The reason for this high rate of edentulousness is that these senior citizens grew up in a time before the benefits of fluoridation and other preventive measures were known. Extraction of teeth—which today is a last resort in most instances—was far more common in the past when alternative tooth-saving procedures were not known. Hence, many of the acute dental problems common to the elderly in the 1970s will become less prevalent in the future. For instance, the National Center for Health Statistics reported that edentulousness among elderly Americans declined significantly between 1958 and 1971. For those between 65 and 74 edentulousness declined by 10 percent, and for those 75 and over the decline was 7.5 percent.

There is also considerable evidence that the rate of edentulousness is still declining steadily. The American Dental Association did a survey in 1960 and found that 31 percent of people between the ages of 30 and 39 were wearing dentures or bridges. A similar survey done in 1975 on the same age group revealed that the rate had declined to 11 percent.

The conditions of the edentulous elderly in the mid-1970s were rather abysmal. It was found that six hundred thousand of the 11.4 million elderly were without any teeth at all—dentures or natural teeth. Another 3.4 million of the elderly had dentures that needed to be replaced or refitted. Another interesting finding revealed by HEW, states that about 1.3 million people over age 65 had so much difficulty wearing these inadequate dentures that they never used them or wore them only part of the time.

This set of statistics clearly shows that large numbers of the elderly are in need of dental care—care of their own natural teeth or of the dentures or bridges they are wearing. These problems are the result of years of inadequate care and are much more serious than those found among the younger population. Yet the elderly use considerably fewer dental services than do the younger segments of the population.

It is important that people who have had their teeth removed be fitted with dentures quickly. If too much time elapses between the teeth removal and the denture fitting, it becomes extremely difficult for the person to adjust to the dentures.

The importance of teeth or dentures is frequently not realized. The nonuse of dentures or the use of faulty dentures frequently means that an elderly person is forced to choose foods that are easier to chew but lower in nutritional value. The edentulous tend to avoid foods like meat, raw vegetables, and fresh fruits because these foods are difficult to chew.

Dental care including the fitting of dentures, is expensive, and this factor frequently inhibits the elderly from obtaining adequate dental care. Costs for obtaining dentures—including the extraction, x-rays, making of impressions, and the purchase of the dentures from the laboratory—can vary from $500 to $1,000. These costs were estimated during the mid-1970s and are clearly higher now.

If the elderly are fortunate enough to live near a dental clinic that specializes in dentures, costs can be reduced substantially. For example, in the mid-1970s the Seaton Clinic in Florence, South Carolina provided dentures for substantially less than the average cost of $500 to over $1,000. Although the South Carolina Dental Association has alleged that they have received numerous complaints from patients of the clinic, the clinic's tremendous volume of business indicates that there must also be a large group of satisfied clients. The author is personally familiar with the dental clinics in Canada's province of Ontario that are frequented by many American residents in border cities such as Buffalo and Detroit. The cost of obtaining dentures through those clinics is frequently only a fraction of what is paid if the dentures are obtained through the services of a local dentist.

These conditions imply that there are considerable economies of scale in providing dentures to people. The economies of scale are not just the result of the higher volume of a clinic versus a dentist office. It appears that the fitting of a denture, including the adjustments to the denture, can be handled more efficiently by the laboratory technician than by the dentist. The dentist's time is more valuable and as a result his or her professional fee will be higher. The dental technician, however, is probably more skilled in fitting and adjusting dentures since that is his or her specialty. (These are hypotheses based on considerable evidence but have not been proven yet.)

It is not quite clear from the evidence whether economies of scale also exist in providing routine dental services to those people who still have all of their teeth. The author believes that there are few economies of scale in providing routine dental care. It is difficult to improve the efficiency of the personal services of a dentist, especially if that dentist is already utilizing dental assistants, dental hygienists, and administrative and clerical support staff.

What this implies, therefore, is that the elderly can expect to gain little in reduced costs if they still have all their teeth and are determined to maintain their teeth. They must seek out dental care and pay the prevailing prices for such care. If, on the other hand, the elderly need dentures, there are ways of obtaining services at lower cost. These services can be obtained at clinics like the ones described above. In those communities where such clinics do not yet exist, there will be increasing pressure to develop such clinics.

RECOMMENDATIONS FOR COST CONTAINMENT

The report of the Subcommittee on Health and Long Term Care contained numerous suggestions on how consumers can avoid overpricing and unnecessary services. In general, the subcommittee recommended that the objective of every consumer should be to obtain the highest possible quality at the lowest possible price. It was also recommended that where appropriate and feasible, government at all levels should make efforts to disseminate as much information as possible to ensure that the people affected can make the correct decisions.

Specifically, in the area of vision care, the consumer is urged to ensure that the eye examination by the optometrist or ophthalmologist is thorough. The consumer should be sure that the health professional takes a complete case history regarding vision and that tests for near, distance, depth, peripheral, color, coordination, and unaided vision are taken. It is also important to be sure that eye charts appear clear and that adequate lighting is available.

Following the eye examination the client should not simply accept what is suggested but should ask questions. The client who already has eyeglasses should ask about the difference between the present glasses and the suggested ones. If the change is small, a second opinion may not be necessary. If it is accepted that new eyeglasses are needed, the client should take the prescription and shop around. There are considerable variations in the cost of eyeglasses.

Similar guidelines also apply in the case of a hearing examination. Before acquiring a hearing aid, the client should have his or her hearing examined by an otolaryngologist or an otologist. Both are physicians and should provide an unbiased evaluation of whether a hearing aid is needed.

After determining that a hearing aid is needed, the consumer should shop around among the many hearing aid dealers. Before purchasing a hearing aid, the customer should check what guarantee comes with the aid. Some dealers offer money back guarantees if a customer is not satisfied. Also check comparisons of hearing aids by such organizations as Consumers' Union, the publishers of *Consumer Reports* magazine.

After purchasing the hearing aid the consumer should follow the manufacturer's instructions. As is true of any external device, it takes time to become used to it. Usually maximum value is obtained only after one has become accustomed to the aid.

The subcommittee also recommended that consumers shop around for dental care, especially for price. Although there is generally uniform pricing among dentists in a community, there always are those who price their services higher or lower than the norm. The consumer should not be afraid to call a dentist and ask how much a given procedure will cost. Price is particularly important in the case of dentures. A local dentist should be consulted first. But the wise consumer also checks dental clinics (independent or associated with dental schools) that might provide dentures at a lower cost. Before making a final decision on complete or partial dentures, the consumer should be sure that everything is spelled out as far as cost, payment, and delivery time is concerned.

CONCLUSIONS

This chapter has explored the delivery systems for eyeglasses, hearing aids, and dentures. Although these three products are used by all age groups, it is the elderly who particularly need these products because they can at least partially alleviate so many disabilities.

Cost is the big barrier to acquiring these products and the services that go along with them. None of these services are fully covered by Medicare, and private health insurance typically does not cover any of these products or services. Medicaid may cover part of these services in some states. Hence, the elderly generally must pay for these products and services out of their current budgets. Unfortunately, most people over age 65 cannot afford the extensive costs involved in the acquisition of eyeglasses, dentures, or hearing aids. So acquisition is postponed or does not occur at all. As a result, the quality of life of many of the elderly is severely reduced, and they suffer feelings of loneliness, degradation, and inferiority.   There are two possible solutions to this situation: (1) develop delivery systems for eyeglasses, hearing aids, and dentures that will cause costs to be reduced substantially, to a level that all elderly could afford; (2) provide total or at least partial coverage for the three products and services under Medicare.

NOTES

1. U.S. House of Representatives, Subcommittee on Health and Long Term Care of the Select Committee on Aging, "Medical Appliances and the Elderly: Unmet Needs and Excessive Costs for Eyeglasses, Hearing Aids, Dentures, and Other Devices " (Washington, D.C.: U.S. Government Printing Office, September 1976).

Chapter 17

Medicare and Its Limitations

M edicare was established in 1965 under Title XVIII of the Social Security Act. Its intent was to ease access to quality health care for the elderly population. In some respects it can be called a form of national health insurance restricted to those age 65 and over.

The origin of Medicare can be traced back to the Kerr-Mills Act of 1960. The benefits that the Kerr-Mills Act secured for the elderly have lent it this distinction. In addition, it puts Medicare into historical perspective—a reflection of federal policies begun in the 1960s aimed at improving the overall quality of life in America. The logic of the Medicare-Medicaid program is that increased accessibility to health care services will result in a healthier population. It is important to note that the extrinsic benefits of better health accorded to this group actually stem from a more basic intrinsic benefit: the establishment of an individual's legal right to health care.

Medicare provides hospitalization and medical insurance for those 65 and over who are eligible for Social Security or railroad retirement benefits. In fiscal 1974 coverage was extended to include younger persons with chronic renal disease and disabled persons who had been receiving Social Security cash benefits for two or more years.

The Medicare program embodies two insurance formats. Hospital Insurance (HI) is Part A of the program and offers a variety of hospital and institutional services. While these benefits are generally more comprehensive than those in comparative private health plans, they are still subject to specified deductible and coinsurance requirements.

Supplemental Medical Insurance (SMI) is Part B of the program, and is a voluntary plan that covers services ancillary to the intensive care of Part A, such as physician services and outpatient hospital services. Unlike Part A, those 65 and older can attain SMI membership even though they are not eligible for Social Security Insurance. Financing of each plan requires input from both the government and the beneficiary. The details of this process are discussed later. Medicare has greatly expanded the role of the federal and state governments in financing and delivering health care services. The program has made substantial progress in making quality health care available to the elderly by reducing financial barriers and thus encouraging utilization.

MEDICARE EXPENDITURES OVER TIME

Medicare has been under close scrutiny in recent years because of the rapid increase in government expenditures for health care and the rapid inflation in health care costs. These factors are pointing out many of the inherent shortcomings that were neglected in the program's inception. The net effect is an imbalance in the present cost-benefit equation and a general erosion of the intrinsic and extrinsic benefits originally offered the beneficiary.

Table 17-1 shows the increase in Medicare expenditures for the years 1967–75. Column 1 illustrates that Medicare expenditures have quadrupled in the eight-year period, from $4,049 million to $14,464 million. More important, column 2, showing the number of people affected, clearly indicates that only 25 percent of this increase is attributable to increased use by the elderly. Therefore, the remaining 75 percent can be traced to inflation in the price of hospital care. The effect of this on Part A of the Medicare plan has been to raise the actual cost per member (column 3) from $152 in fiscal 1967 to $442 in fiscal 1975. In constant 1967 dollars (column 5) these totals were only $152 and $186 respectively.

Similarly, the increase in total Medicare expenditures attributable to SMI has been largely inflationary. Expenditures increased 243 percent, but only one third of this total is due to increased membership. Since SMI payments are generally put toward physician vendor reimbursement, it is clear that most of the inflation can be traced to a rise in physicians' fees. Also note that in constant 1967 dollars, hospital insurance increased 22 percent while SMI payments increased 58 percent during the 1967–1975 period on a per person basis.

Obviously, the rise in government expenditures for Medicare is inexorably linked to rampant inflation in the cost of health care, rather than to a comparable increase in the output of services. The tragedy of this vicious circle can be seen most explicitly as it affects the individual beneficiary.

WHAT DOES MEDICARE COVER?

When discussing what Medicare covers we must first specify Part A or Part B because Medicare consists of two parts. The hospital insurance portion, usually referred to as Part A, stipulates the following payment provisions for a given benefit period. The plan covers:

Table 17-1 Summary of Hospital Insurance and Supplemental Medical Insurance Under Medicare, Fiscal Years 1967–75

Year	1 Expenditures (millions of dollars)	2 Number of people* (millions)	3 Expenditures per person (dollars)	4 Related consumer price index** (1967 = 100)	5 Expenditures per person (1967 dollars)
Hospital Insurance (HI)					
1967	$2,886	19.0	$152	100.0	$152
1968	3,841	19.4	198	115.9	171
1969	4,641	19.6	236	131.5	179
1970	4,992	19.9	250	148.3	169
1971	5,602	20.3	276	168.0	164
1972	6,161	20.6	299	183.8	163
1973	6,743	20.9	322	193.0	167
1974	8,201	23.1	355	204.6	174
1975	10,471	23.7	442	238.2	186
Supplementary Medical Insurance (SMI)					
1967	1,163	17.8	66	100.0	66
1968	1,490	18.0	83	106.1	78
1969	1,748	18.8	93	112.6	83
1970	1,896	19.3	98	120.7	81
1971	2,072	19.7	105	129.8	81
1972	2,299	20.0	115	136.5	84
1973	2,454	20.4	120	140.0	86
1974	3,256	22.6	144	147.0	98
1975	3,993	23.2	172	165.8	104
Addenda					
Percent Increase, 1967–75					
HI	263	25	191	138	22
SMI	243	30	161	66	58

* For HI, number of people eligible; for SMI, number of people enrolled.
** For HI the consumer price index is based on semiprivate hospital rooms. For SMI the consumer price index is based on physicians' fees.
Source: K. Davis and C. Schoen, *Health and the War on Poverty* (Washington, D.C.: The Brookings Institutions, 1978), p. 98.

1. full costs of inpatient hospital services for 60 days; the beneficiary pays a deductible equal to the cost of approximately one day of hospital care.
2. 75 percent of inpatient hospital services between the sixty-first and ninetieth days; the beneficiary pays the remaining 25 percent.
3. 50 percent of inpatient hospital services between the ninety-first and one hundred and fiftieth day; the beneficiary pays the remaining 50 percent.

Table 17-2 Hospital Insurance Deductible and Coinsurance Payments by Beneficiaries Under Medicare

Number of Days	Type Payment	Hospital Insurance				Percent Increase 1966–78
		1966	1976	1977	1978	
1–60	*Deductible	$40	$104	$124	$144	277%
61–90	**Coinsurance (per day)	10	26	31	36	277%
91–150	Coinsurance	20	52	62	72	277%

* Deductible—amount paid by patient before insurance benefits begin.
** Coinsurance—cost-sharing percentage of total medical bill paid by the patient after meeting the deductible.
Source: Social Security Bulletin, 40, 7 (July 1978).

What this government payment schedule means to the individual in terms of required payments is illustrated in Table 17-2.

The dollar figures in Table 17-2 represent actual out-of-pocket expenses that the elderly must pay for hospitalization, and they show a 277 percent increase between 1966 and 1978. Because of these deductible and coinsurance provisions, more than one half of Americans age 65 and over are now buying private insurance to supplement Medicare. Premiums for this insurance cost the elderly several billion dollars annually.

Table 17-2 shows that a large share of the financial burden of hospitalization is being passed on to the aged. This is a very important point because, as will be shown later, the Medicare program itself is partly responsible for the inflationary dilemma.

Table 17-3 breaks down the inflationary spiral on a per person basis. Part One concentrates on increases in the cost of health services by five categories. While the acceleration in each category is certainly dramatic, it must be remembered that part of the increase is due to higher utilization of these services by the elderly population. For example, after Medicare went into effect, the use of health services by those age 65 and over jumped 25 percent.

The greater quantity of health care services available to the elderly under Medicare has apparently led to a parallel development in the quality of these services. General qualitative improvements have been most apparent in the area of extended care and home health services, both of which barely existed before Medicare. Also, for people age 65 and over, discharges from short-term hospitals per 100 persons per annum rose from 17.0 in 1962 to 23.8 in 1973, an increase of 40 percent. In the same period the elderly had 15 percent fewer days

Table 17-3 Per Capita Personal Health Care Expenditures For Persons 65 and Over

Part One—By Type of Service*

Health Care Category	1966	1967	1976
Hospital Care	$177.84	$197.63	$688.59
Physician's Services	89.57	108.97	255.97
Nursing Home	68.39	89.94	350.61
Drugs	62.40	67.57	121.22
Other Medical Services	47.06	49.98	105.01
Total Expenditures	$445.25	$509.09	$1521.36

Part Two—Percentage Distribution by Payment Source**

Payment Source	1966	1967	1976
Private	69	40	32
Public (largely Medicaid)	31	26	25
Medicare	0	34	43
Total	100	100	100

* *Source: Health U.S., 1966–1977*, U.S. Department of Health, Education and Welfare (Washington, D.C.: U.S. Government Printing Office, 1977).

** *Sources: Medical Care Chart Book*, Bureau of Public Health Economics (Ann Arbor, Michigan: University of Michigan, 1972), p. 283. Also *Trends Affecting U.S. Health Care System*, U.S. Department of Health, Education and Welfare (Washington, D.C.: U.S. Government Printing Office, 1976). And *Social Security Bulletin* 40, no. 6 (June 1977), and *Social Security Bulletin* 40, no. 8 (August 1977).

of restricted activity, the limitation of activity caused by chronic conditions declined, and mortality rates were lower than might have been predicted from previous experience.[1]

The cost associated with these improvements in quality and quantity is broken down in Part Two of Table 17-3. Part Two converts the total expenditures to a percentage distribution by payment source. As illustrated, there was growth in the proportion of the total bill paid out of Medicare, from 34 percent to 43 percent.

STRUCTURAL LIMITATIONS OF MEDICARE

By this point it should be apparent that, regardless of certain accomplishments, Medicare coverage has fallen short of goals in many areas. This was formally recognized as early as 1966 in U.S. Senate hearings that criticized the program's reimbursement formula for paying doctors and hospitals (1966), its role in financing teaching hospitals (1969), its efficiency (1970), and finally made overall suggestions for improvement (1970).

In all fairness, the purpose of these hearings was to attack the problems of Medicare, rather than to attack the program itself. For example, one senator remarked that "Medicare has proven to be a most important element contributing to security of our aged citizens. It has permitted them to enjoy their twilight years in dignity and with less fear that illness will drain their financial resources." [2] Still one cannot ignore the system's deficiencies.

In the broadest sense, there appear to be two key problems in the Medicare dilemma: (1) provisions of the program that give rise to inflationary pressures in the cost of health care; (2) inadequate protection. However, a network of specific catalysts underlie these broad problems, and each merits some degree of blame as a limitation that mars the total system.

The most significant of these limitations was the decision, made at the outset, not to initiate reforms of the health care system or to control costs and promote efficiency. Rather, Medicare joined private health insurance in contributing to the spiraling costs of health care.[3] In the absence of early reforms and limits, Medicare reinforced the existing system of delivering care, including the defects in the system. For example, payment is made through "intermediaries" and "carriers" on the basis of what is "usual, customary, and prevailing." This produced a financing response that lacked cost control measures; it did not restrain the use of high-cost facilities and services when other less expensive alternatives were available.[4]

LIMITATIONS CAUSED BY INFLATIONARY EFFECTS

Another fundamental defect that is directly related to the inflationary effects of Medicare was the early decision to charge a universal positive price to all beneficiaries. Such an approach led to a suboptimal pattern of consumption due to overusage and underusage of services. Overusage arises when individuals consume care whose marginal cost exceeds the value that all persons, including the individual, place on additional units of care. Underusage, on the other hand, may occur in cases associated with premature dismissal from the hospital. Table 17-2 shows that individuals must start coinsurance payments for hospitalization after a stay of 60 days and must pay the full price of care after 150 days. In many instances, this either compels the individual to skimp on this care or face financial ruin.

If the out-of-pocket price is set at a level that ensures that middle-income individuals use the optimal amount of care, there will be underconsumption of care by low-income individuals and overconsumption of care by high-income individuals. In the case of Medicare, the price was put at a level that induced low-income individuals to use an optimal amount of care, with the predictable result being an increased use of services at all income levels. Accordingly, this means that some of the additional usage (i.e., middle/high income levels) represents overusage. Not only is this suboptimal (because it encourages usage that far exceeds its benefits), it also contributes to higher expenditures and price inflation. This defect in efficiency could have been cured by a "variable-subsidy" or "progressive premium" format based on some schedule of income.[5]

So far, this section on limitations has discussed Medicare's three basic contributions to the inflationary spiral of medical costs: (1) suboptimal utilization of scarce medical resources, (2) the provision of incentives for the use of the highest cost facilities, and (3) the lack of effective cost control measures. The inflationary pressure that has been generated exists at cross-purposes with the program's original intent. For example, since the introduction of Medicare in 1965, the daily cost of hospital care has increased at an annual rate of about 14 percent, up from about 7 percent during the preceding 10 years. This already severe situation is compounded by the fact that Medicare contributes less than half of the total health bill for those 65 and over. Therefore, after supplying so much fuel to the inflationary fire, Medicare has put some of the elderly at the mercy of higher out-of-pocket costs through inadequate coverage in many crucial areas.

More clearly, the elderly presently pay more for health care (either directly or through insurance premiums) than they did before Medicare and Medicaid ($537 per annum fiscal year 1975 versus $312 fiscal year 1966).[6] Also, a large portion of the rise in aggregate medical care prices since the introduction of the program is due to the program itself. While the benefits made available under Part A (Hospital Insurance) have kept pace with inflation to protect the elderly from the rising cost of hospital care, there are still many areas of medical necessity that are not met by the program. Therefore, financial ruin due to health care expenditures is still a real threat for a considerable percentage of the elderly population.

Another important limitation of Medicare coverage is in the area of nursing home care. The program's failure to grapple with the need for long-term institutional care for those elderly who are unable to care for themselves has resulted in Medicaid becoming responsible for the financing of most nursing home care. Finally, other limitations in Medicare coverage are in prescription drugs and "other medical services" such as dentist's services, hearing aids, and eyeglasses. The combined expenses of these services comprise 15 percent of total 1976 health care expenditures by the aged.[7]

EQUITY LIMITATIONS OF MEDICARE

The limitations discussed thus far have been major structural imbalances and areas of inadequate coverage; the combined effect of these has been to limit the

punch of Medicare legislation, dilute its accomplishments, and leave its beneficiaries liable in many areas of health coverage. However, there is another broad
category of limitations ancillary to these considerations, termed "equity" implications.

Equity implications refer to the distribution of Medicare payments across the
vast subcategories of beneficiaries. The previous discussion treated this group
as a largely homogeneous body on which both the pros and cons of Medicare's
history have had equal effects for all members. However, this assumption ig-
nores the social imbalances that are reflected in the elderly population, and
these must be addressed in order to recognize secondary limitations in access to
Medicare coverage.

The first equity implication is related to income. Simple logic dictates that
the out-of-pocket coinsurance and deductible cost of Medicare coverage rests
heavier on low-income elderly and can often lead to their underutilization in
many uncovered areas. For example, the $98.40 SMI premium in 1978 de-
terred four hundred sixty thousand elderly persons from obtaining this coverage.[8] Because of this situation, it might be generally stated that utilization of
health services still depends to an extent on income rather than needs, and that
Medicare has only reinforced this trend.

The second major equity implication centers on differences in Medicare coverage by location. In general, rural areas have less hospital facilities available,
and those that are available are not always easily accessible. This is important,
as the accessibility of medical care resources to the population—including both
distance and travel time—is often suggested as a factor that affects the use of
services.[9]

Table 17-4 demonstrates this by using "mean length of stay" and "discharges per 1,000 enrollees" as measures of hospital utilization. Part One ranks
the Northeast and North Central regions as the greatest consumers of hospital
services by length of stay; the rural South and West lag far behind. This imbalance is fortified in Part Two: the Northeast has the lowest discharge rate per
1,000 enrollees, and the rural South has the highest. Therefore, with population
held constant, it seems that the Northeastern beneficiary is getting a lot more
hospital coverage under Medicare than his or her Southern counterpart. Since,
over time, this expense to Medicare is reflected in increased out-of-pocket expenses passed on to the beneficiaries, the rural recipients are in effect subsidiz-
ing the urban beneficiaries because premium payments are uniform.

This geographic difference also holds true in the case of SMI benefits. As
mentioned earlier, Medicare reimburses physicians on the basis of local prevailing charges. Physicians in low-income areas charge lower fees, whereas physicians in high-income areas charge higher fees. Since low-income areas tend to
be rural, and high-income areas urban, the concentration of physicians has been

Table 17-4 Geographic Variance of Hospital Stay by Medicare Enrollees

Part One: Mean Length of Stay (in days)

Region	1967	1973	Rank 1967, 1973
United States	13.8	11.8	—
Northeast	16.1	14.3	1
North Central	14.6	12.2	2
South	12.3	10.8	3
West	11.8	9.5	4

Part Two: Discharges per 1,000 Enrollees

United States	261.7	304.6	—
Northeast	217.4	261.0	4
North Central	276.6	320.8	2
South	282.9	328.6	1
West	267.7	299.9	3

Source: Social Security Bulletin 40, no. 6 (June 1977).

toward urban areas. This pattern often makes physician services inaccessible in rural areas, leading to lower utilization. Ironically, Medicare's policy of reimbursement rewards physicians for practicing in areas where physicians are fairly abundant.

CONCLUSIONS

Medicare has been responsible for many positive developments in the delivery of quality health care. But Medicare's goal of helping the elderly gain adequate health care has been circumvented in many areas. The limitations covered in this paper include inflationary structural defects, areas of inadequate coverage, and equity implications in the distribution of services to beneficiaries. This is not to say that Medicare has not made progress towards its goal.

Also, in all fairness it must be remembered that the rising cost of health care can be traced to a combination of factors including: (1) increases in the cost of inputs that go toward producing the service, and (2) changes in the service itself over time to upgrade the quality of care. The analysis in this chapter focused only on the first category of inflation; in cases of the second category, quality changes should be factored out in estimates of inflation.

NOTES

1. U.S. Department of Health, Education and Welfare, *Trends Affecting U.S. Health Care System* (Washington, D.C.: U.S. Government Printing Office, 1976).
2. U.S. Senate, *Hearings Before the Committee on Finance,* February 25 and 26, 1970 (Washington, D.C.: U.S. Government Printing Office, 1970).
3. U.S. Department of Health, Education and Welfare, *Towards a Comprehensive Health Policy,* A White Paper (Washington, D.C.: U.S. Government Printing Office, 1971).
4. Social Security Administration, *Problems Associated with Reimbursements to Hospitals for Services Furnished under Medicare,* Report to the U.S. Congress, U.S. Department of Health, Education and Welfare (Washington, D.C.: U.S. Government Printing Office, 1972).
5. M. J. Pauly, *Medical Care at Public Expense: A Study in Applied Welfare Economics* (New York: Praeger Publishers, *1972), p. 113.*
6. *Health U.S., 1978,* U.S. Department of Health, Education and Welfare (Washington, D.C.: U.S. Government Printing Office, 1978).
7. *Social Security Bulletin* 40, no. 8 (August 1977).
8. Ibid., p. 15.
9. *Social Security Bulletin* 40, no. 6 (June 1977).

Chapter 18

Supplementary Health Insurance and Prepaid Care

O n the average, and in the aggregate, Americans spend about 9 percent of the Gross National Product on health care. However, older Americans spend as much as 30 percent of their income for health care services. A single expenditure of 30 percent imposes a considerable burden on those elderly who make ends meet on a retirement income. When Medicare was established in the 1960s it covered most of the health care costs of the elderly. Since then considerable restrictions have been placed on what Medicare covers. As a result, the elderly incur considerable out-of-pocket expenses for their health maintenance.

In response, an entire new industry has developed to provide supplementary health insurance to the elderly. This insurance covers all or part of the portion that is not covered by Medicare. This chapter reviews the pitfalls and problems with supplementary health insurance.

In addition, another kind of organization is entering the supplementary health insurance market for the elderly. That organization is the Health Maintenance Organization (HMO). The HMO not only provides supplementary health insurance but also delivers a complete range of health care services including those covered, and paid for, by Medicare.

HMOs, with their emphasis on prevention and health maintenance, have most recently been proclaimed as the answer to the spiraling cost of health care. Although not originally developed as a way to provide health care for the elderly, HMOs are now being seen in such a light. This chapter also examines how HMOs came into being, their development, and how they differ from traditional health insurance.

MEDICARE AND MEDICAID PROGRAMS

The Medicare and Medicaid programs have helped senior citizens carry some of this health care cost burden. Government expenditures for these two programs have increased from $9.9 billion in 1970 to about $37 billion in 1977. Taken together, the two programs account for about two-thirds of the average per capita health care costs incurred by the elderly. Precisely, in 1977 government programs paid $1,175 of the $1,739 in per capita health care expenditures for the elderly. The remaining one-third, $564 per person, was paid out-of-pocket by the elderly.[1]

However, these figures are only average figures. Remember, too, that not all older individuals are eligible for both Medicare and Medicaid. Medicaid, which is essentially a welfare program, is only available to about one out of five senior citizens, those whose incomes fall below the poverty line. Individuals with incomes over $3000 per year are generally not eligible for Medicaid. For those not covered by Medicaid, Medicare covers only 38 percent of the average senior's yearly health care bill.

Medicaid is generally thought of as a welfare program by most of the population. As a result, having to accept Medicaid is a traumatic occasion for the vast majority of senior citizens who have grown up believing that one must care for oneself and not be dependent on government handouts. Interestingly enough, there is virtually no trauma associated with having to accept government help through Medicare. Medicare reimbursement, with all its limitations, is considered to be a civil right.

SUPPLEMENTARY HEALTH INSURANCE

In order to offset the ever-escalating cost of health care, senior citizens are buying private health insurance policies to supplement their Medicare coverage. Two-thirds, or 15 million of 23 million older Americans, have at least one such policy. These policies are often called "wraparound" (around Medicare) health insurance or "medigap" insurance. Senior citizens often acquire more than one such policy and often have as many as four or five. As of 1978, there were an estimated 19 million health insurance policies in effect for the elderly.

Seniors pay an average of $200 in annual premiums for each policy—a total expenditure of $3.8 billion. The policyholders received an estimated $1.3 billion in benefits, which amounts to less than 35 percent of premiums collected.

The low return on these health insurance policies is in part caused by the fact that many elderly hold multiple policies in order to maximize protection. However, when they become sick, they can usually only claim on one policy. The real beneficiaries of this wasteful practice are the private insurance companies who reimburse claims on one policy at most. Private health insurance has about 50 percent of the elderly health insurance market. Blue Cross/Blue Shield and HMOs cover the balance. None of the practices described here are attributed to these latter organizations.

It is in the sector, involving the private insurance companies that sell to individuals, that most problems have occurred. A congressional investigation decided that the root of the problem lies in the limited coverage that Medicare provides and in the inability of many older Americans to understand what Medicare covers.

Before analyzing supplementary health insurance, it is useful to examine HMOs, their history, their rapid growth, and their special importance for the elderly in the future.

THE HEALTH MAINTENANCE ORGANIZATION

How Does the HMO Differ From Traditional Health Insurance?

McNeil and Schlenker[2] define HMOs as

> an organization which accepts contractual responsibility to assure the delivery of a stated range of health services, including at least ambulatory and in-hospital care to a voluntarily enrolled population in exchange for an advance capitation payment where the organization assumes at least part of the financial risk or shares in the surplus associated with the delivery of medical services.

Traditional health insurance is dominated by what is commonly termed the "exclusion mentality." That is, certain types of services are excluded, and many services are usually restricted to treatment of illnesses. Preventive care and routine medical checkups are seldom included. As a result, the individual must be ill before medical assistance can be reimbursed.

The other more subtle difference is in the delivery of health care. The HMO delivers health care for a prepaid fee. Health insurance reimburses only if a claim is filed by or on behalf of the insured individual.

Both HMOs and health insurers would benefit from a public more informed about healthful living. However, the HMO, by promoting preventive health maintenance, has been the more active of the two in educating its membership about the benefits of proper nutrition, and the dangers of alcohol, tobacco, and stressful living.

History of HMOs

Organizations that provide a broad range of medical services for a prepaid monthly fee have been around for a long time. Around the turn of the century a group that provided prepaid health care was established in San Francisco.

The major movement in America for prepaid health care can be traced back to the Kaiser Foundation Health Plan, more commonly known as Kaiser Permanente. The Kaiser organization retained a small group of doctors to provide health care to Kaiser employees who were working on a large-scale construction project on the Mojave Desert. The plan gradually expanded to cover workers at other Kaiser locations and was opened to the public after World War II. The Kaiser Foundation Health Plan now has about 25 hospitals and 60 medical centers serving about 3.3 million members in California, Oregon, Hawaii, Washington, Ohio, and Colorado. Its membership accounts for 40 percent of a total HMO population of nearly 9 million people.

Growth in HMO organizations has been intensive in recent years because of federal support for their development. About 200 organizations are currently operational. Most of these have just recently been started; still others are in the preoperational stages.

HMO Development

In the past, successful functioning of at least one HMO in an urban area has resulted in the formation of other HMOs. Although they may compete against one another to some extent, the presence of several HMOs in a given metropolitan area provides competition for the major health insurers in that area. This phenomenon, in turn, creates a considerable economic force that keeps the costs of hospital and other health services at a reasonable level. To illustrate, there are now eight operational HMOs in the Minneapolis metropolitan area. HMO enrollment in the Minneapolis area is growing at an aggregate rate of fifty thousand members per year, and it is projected that soon the majority of residents will be members of one of the HMOs. Coincidentally, health care costs in the Minneapolis area are among the lowest of this country's larger metropolitan areas. Although, the HMOs cannot take credit for this condition, their presence does guarantee that health care costs in Minneapolis will remain reasonable in relation to those in other metropolitan areas.

Just how HMOs can promise to control costs can be revealed by examining their distinctly different development in comparison to traditional health insurance.

Traditional health insurance reimburses the insured for health care costs incurred. The insurance carriers usually have little control over costs and utilization of health care services. As a result, traditional health insurance is largely a payment mechanism to finance health care and especially hospital-based health care.

HMOs on the other hand, not only provide health insurance but also provide or arrange for provision of the health care services. In addition, HMOs provide much more comprehensive coverage of health services than those provided by the typical health insurance.

Since HMOs provide more comprehensive coverage and at the same time compete with traditional health insurance, they have a strong incentive to contain costs. Cost containment is attained by lower hospitalization rates for HMO members. The savings obtained from lower hospitalization are then available to provide more comprehensive health care in such areas as ambulatory care, drug therapy, physical therapy and others.

HMOs and the Elderly

HMOs have wide appeal for all segments of the population, but there are certain specific health care needs of the elderly that make HMOs an especially attractive alternative for them. First, HMOs bring various medical specialties together under one roof. Because elderly people are likely to suffer from multiple symptoms and various interrelated disabilities, HMOs may reduce the transportation costs of medical care and the bother and frustrations that often go along with these extra costs. Second, elderly people may feel uncomfortable about seeking a second opinion on a medical problem. When dealing with HMOs there is no need to seek a second opinion because medical histories are regularly brought to the attention of other doctors at staff meetings. Third, when older persons move, they must find a new physician. Through HMO membership the availability of physicians is assured, and HMO physicians are those whose qualifications are under continuous review by their peers. Finally, there is the issue of cost. Cost is probably the central factor that makes the elderly opt for this type of health care delivery. The HMO, with a provision for prepayment, enables older people to budget their expenses and be protected against the threat of catastrophic illness. The vast majority of today's elderly live on fixed incomes. Alleviating this threat may in turn alleviate the fears and anxiety that can contribute to illness.

At present, the Social Security Administration, the agency that administers Medicare, only partially allows prepayment plans for the elderly who choose to join HMOs. It is anticipated, however that this policy will change soon, making HMOs available to the elderly in those areas of the country where they have become operational.

Recent studies by the Social Security Administration have shown that the costs incurred by Medicare for services to its aged beneficiaries enrolled in HMOs were significantly lower than for comparable elderly persons receiving care in the open medical market. The data were drawn from six geographic areas throughout the nation. For HMO members, the aggregate costs of physician services to ambulatory patients and of home health services were higher. But the aggregate costs of expensive inpatient hospital and nursing home services were so much lower that the overall expenditures for HMO members were lower.

Although this finding is impressive, there are still difficulties in assessing the value of HMOs because of the lack of baseline data. Only about 1.5 percent of Medicare beneficiaries participate in HMOs. Most of these enrollees were already in HMOs prior to their eligibility for Medicare. Thus little is known about HMOs in relation to individuals who join for the first time during their old age.

This lack of knowledge about HMOs is perhaps the reason why current restrictions in the Medicare Act prevent eligibles from fully participating in HMOs. For instance, Medicare's reimbursement policy under Section 1833 does not provide an advance capitation rate, will not reimburse for services that are made available but not used, does not cover comprehensive range of health services, and provides no financial incentives for an organization to keep costs low or to control utilization of services by its Medicare beneficiaries.

Through enactment of Section 1876 of the Social Security Act, it has been dictated that at least half of the enrolled membership of an HMO must be under 65, and membership must be representative of the population in the enrollment area. An additional roadblock dictates that once an individual is enrolled in an HMO under Medicare, the HMO must provide care for at least one year. Thus the beneficiary is "locked in" to the plan, and only care provided by the HMO will be reimbursed by Medicare.

All of this means that HMOs will definitely have a future impact on the delivery of health care to the elderly. This care will be comprehensive, including not only those procedures covered by Medicare but also those procedures and services not covered by Medicare but typically paid for directly by the patient or covered by private medigap health insurance. Below we shall analyze in more detail the health insurance needs of the elderly as they exist today.

HOW SUPPLEMENTARY HEALTH INSURANCE MEETS THE NEEDS OF THE ELDERLY

Critics of supplemental insurance, especially that provided by private health insurance plans, know that no insurance policy will cover everything that Medicare does not cover. Some items that are frequently excluded from supplemental policies are: private duty nursing, routine checkups, eyeglasses, hearing aids, dental work, cosmetic surgery, custodial care in nursing homes, psychiatric care, and self-administered drugs. Most supplemental policies also follow Medicare guidelines. This fact more than any other causes one to question why such policies are needed at all.

Senior citizens naively purchase these supplementary policies with the hope and expectations that they will cover all of the medical expenses not covered by

Medicare. Insurance agents often assure their prospective customers that their policy does provide this coverage. In reality, however, the holder of numerous policies often discovers too late that the policies do not provide the security that they sought.

Although the case of the individual who holds numerous policies paints a shady view of the insurance industry as a whole, most experts agree that there is good economic value and reasonable financial risk protection in purchasing one supplementary health insurance policy, particularly from a reputable organization such as Blue Cross/Blue Shield. Blue Cross/Blue Shield and other reputable private insurance companies return to the insured in some cases more than 90 percent of the premiums collected in the form of claims paid. On the other hand, there are many other private insurance companies that sell policies that return as little as 20 percent of premiums collected.[3] It is these private insurance companies that give a bad name to the insurance industry as a whole.

Excessive Supplemental Coverage

A report by the Federal Trade Commission states that one-quarter of the elderly Americans who annually spend billions for extra insurance to cover Medicare gaps actually buy unnecessary, costly, and overlapping coverage.[4] The report goes on to say that a lack of consumer information, unscrupulous sales tactics by some firms, and a lack of uniformity in policies has created considerable confusion among consumers and has contributed to higher health care costs for elderly persons living on fixed incomes.

Of all the sales techniques used by insurance agents, perhaps the most unscrupulous and the most effective is the use of scare tactics. It is easy for agents to prey on senior citizens' fears concerning failing health. Typically, they speak about older persons getting sick or ending up dependent on relatives. Many elderly individuals have ample coverage, but there are insurance agents who will always find an excuse to convince the senior citizen to buy more insurance, irrespective of how much coverage that person already has. They will either suggest replacing a current policy with what they claim is a better policy with another company, or sell the individual an additional (and usually unnecessary) policy. Reports have indicated that some persons hold as many as 10 or 12 different health insurance policies—and spend $2,000 or $3,000 a year in health care premiums.

One case history illustrates the extent of this fraudulent activity: One 92-year-old victim in Dallas, Texas was solicited for insurance 13 times between April 1972 and July 1974. She paid $3,440 by checks plus $1,000 in cash and received nothing in return. On April 16, 1974, she paid $975 on an insurance pitch that would allegedly combine and pay up her accident and health policies. She allegedly was to begin receiving $100 per month from paid-up insurance.

However, the money went to purchase a worthless vehicle warranty, even though she did not own an automobile.

A review of numerous other cases reveals that elderly persons tend to be timid and trusting, unsophisticated in the ways of confidence men, and vulnerable to the high-pressure tactics used by dishonest promoters. Investigations also indicate that in addition to selling fraudulent policies, some salesmen overcharged their victims and even resorted to forgery to obtain applications.

Fraudulent Practices

A 1972 investigation by Pennsylvania Insurance Commissioner Herbert S. Denenberg[5,6] revealed the following fraudulent practices by health insurance companies—especially mail order insurance companies:

1. *Insurance companies offer narrow and limited coverage but make it sound liberal.* Typically, an advertisement may proclaim that the company offers $50,000 in benefits, but what it really offers is about $20 a day if, and only if, a claimant is in a hospital. In order to collect $50,000 a person must need continuous hospitalization for about 5 years—a virtual impossibility. According to the extensive experience of one Blue Cross plan, only two percent of all hospitalized people require stays of longer than 30 days.
2. *The insurance companies make sure premiums are used up in expenses and especially profits.* One company returned only 27 cents on each premium dollar and reached profits of up to 46.5 percent on one series of policies.
3. *Insurance companies use scare tactics.* An effective tactic is to push the idea that present coverage is not enough. Agents try to convince prospective clients that hospital costs are skyrocketing and therefore their coverage is insufficient. The bold advertising headlines of mail order operators suggest to seniors that they must have health insurance or they will die in the pauper's ward. Or the advertising may remind them that they certainly don't want to be a burden to their relatives and children.

CONCLUSIONS

Medicare was originally designed as a national health insurance program for the elderly. Financed by employers, by employee contributions, and by the government, its intent was that Americans would draw on this "trust" for their health care costs when they reached age 65. In its early days of operation, Medicare paid about 50 percent of the average senior's total health care bill. But by 1978, Medicare only paid about 38 percent. What contributed to this reduced coverage is the decreasing number of physicians who agree to accept what Medicare pays as full and final payment for services rendered. In 1978 only 50 percent of physicians (as compared to 66 percent in the early days of Medicare) were accepting Medicare reimbursements as full payment. Doctors instead chose to charge the patient a greater amount, and then let the patient worry about being reimbursed from Medicare. Any extra charges over and above what Medicare recognizes as a reasonable charge had to be paid by the patient.

Health maintenance organizations avoid these conditions. Unfortunately, HMOs were developed chiefly to provide an alternative form of comprehensive health care for the under-65 population. But more and more this form of health care is being considered as an alternative for the elderly. Although the Social Security Administration has not given HMOs its full support, there are indications that it will do so in the near future. When this happens the elderly will be able to opt for HMO membership, and will thus be able to gain much improved access to a wider range of health care services, ranging from ambulatory to institutional care.

For the majority of seniors, HMOs are not yet a viable alternative. For them, the purchase of health insurance to supplement Medicare seems to be the only answer. However, as most seniors find out, these policies are very limited in scope. In 1978 about 15 million older Americans, or two-thirds of our 23 million seniors, had at least one supplemental policy. The number of policies held by the elderly has increased 45 percent since 1972, and since that year the cost of these policies has increased more than sevenfold, to $3.8 billion in 1978.

Despite these figures, only six states have instituted specific regulations addressed to abuses in the sale of medigap insurance. The federal government also has been lax in regulating insurance companies that specialize in sales to the elderly. By virtue of the McCarran-Ferguson Act of 1945, Congress delegated federal responsibility for the regulation of insurance to the states. Now, with the advent of National Health Insurance, the federal government again has the opportunity to come to the rescue of victims of a colossal racket that has gone unnoticed and largely unregulated for years.

NOTES

1. "Abuses in the Sale of Health Insurance to the Elderly in Supplementation of Medicare: A National Scandal," A Staff Study by the Select Committee on Aging (Washington D.C.: U.S. Government Printing Office, 1978).

2. R. McNeil, Jr. and R. E. Schlenker, "HMOs Competition and Government," *Millbank Memorial Fund Quarterly (MMFQ)/Health and Society* (Spring 1975): 195-224.

3. P. Gaines, Jr., "77 Claims Ratio Favored," *The National Underwriter*, Vol. 82, no. 24, June 17, 1978, p. 1.

4. "Abuses in the Sale of Health Insurance to the Elderly in Supplementation of Medicare: A National Scandal," 1978.

5. Hearings of the Senate Judiciary Committee's Subcommittee on Anti-Trust and Monopoly, Summer 1972.

6. Herbert S. Denenberg, "Those Health Insurance Booby Traps," *The Progressive* (September 1972): 29-33.

Chapter 19

Quality and Cost Containment Efforts

T he quality of medical care is an issue that has been receiving more and more public attention because of the occasional Medicare or Medicaid scandal that surfaces in the media. It is likely that this issue will continue to arouse public feelings. One critical concern is the role of federal and state governments in setting and enforcing regulations and in defining the minimum criteria of care. The dual role the federal government performs in programs such as Medicaid is often overlooked: (1) the government finances over 50 percent of the care delivered in nursing homes, and (2) the government regulates the quality of that care. The conflict is self-evident. Any commitment to improve standards relating to quality involves a commitment to finance at least part of the subsequent increase in cost.[1]

REIMBURSEMENT TIED TO CONTROLS

For the above reason, state and federal legislators have been developing packages of reimbursement and control mechanisms related to nursing home care. They hope that these package plans simultaneously encourage efficiency and effectiveness of service. However, an appropriate balancing policy of reimbursement has been an elusive goal. At best, legislators have been able to achieve short-term objectives, whether the goal is quality or cost reduction, depending on the social preference or pressures of the time. Social reform and quality were the important issues of the Sixties. The Seventies turned into an era of pulling in the reins on the enormous financial liabilities incurred by previous social goals. It seems certain that in the early Eighties reducing the costs of care will continue to be the more dominant goal.

Below are the two vehicles by which the federal government and State and local governments participate in the cost-reimbursement process. The first vehicle is Medicaid; the second is Medicare.

MEDICAID PROGRAM COSTS

Medicaid is the most prominent of the two federal cost-reimbursement programs. Because of its vast size and its enormous cost to federal, state, and local governments, it has been under close scrutiny by the press, by other public media, and also by the U.S. Congress and its special committees. To give the reader an understanding of the Medicaid reimbursement process and also the involvement of Congress, this chapter features excerpts of testimony before the U.S. Senate Subcommittee on Long-Term care of the Special Committee on the Aging.[2] The testimony concentrates on New York State's method of reimbursement, but it is typical of problems faced by officials in other states as well. New York's method of reimbursement at that time was more sophisticated than that of most other states. New York State's Medicaid Reimbursement formula is shown in Figure 19-1. Modified excerpts of the testimony by Mr. Moan, a New York State official, follow below and explain this figure.

The HE-2 (Operator's Statement of Cost) is a form which is certified by a CPA, and it is verified by the operators as being true and accurate, and a false statement on these applications would be the same thing as perjury under oath.

The various costs are limited according to certain formulas. The first costs to consider are the administration costs.

Administration costs is comprised of the operator's income, what the nursing home operator—the owner—pays himself as a salary.

All figures are subject to dollar maximums, the dollar maximums are calculated by the State Department of Health, and they vary according to the size of the nursing home. For instance, a 100-bed nursing home will have a maximum administrator's salary of $25,000 and a 250-bed nursing home will have a maximum salary of $45,000. The dollar maximum limits the actual dollar amounts that can be charged by the administrator.

The next category is salaries and administrative costs other than the administrator's salary. This category excludes nurses but includes advisors such as legal and accounting.

Other categories are dietary and food costs, laundry, linen and housekeeping costs; and real property costs.

Real property costs are based upon one of two things. If it is a rent situation, it is based upon rent. If it is an ownership situation, where the owner of the nursing home actually owns the building that he is occupying as a business, then this will be included as a depreciation cost.

Figure 19-1 New York State Medicaid Reimbursement Formula

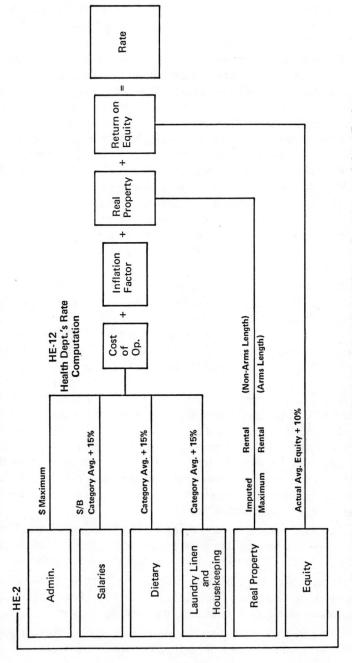

Source: U.S. Senate Subcommittee on Long–Term Care of the Special Senate Committee on Aging, "Testimony on Medicaid Reimbursement Process," January 21, 1975.

The last category is an equity category; that is, how much equity is left in the business at the end of the year. Profit allowed in the business is based on the equity the owner has in the business. The larger the equity, the larger is the profit allowed.

The maximum reimbursement for the other categories—salaries, dietary, and housekeeping—is not limited by dollar amounts. It is limited by the category average plus 15 percent. Category average is determined by the size of the nursing home. For example, nursing homes in New York City from 50 to 150 beds are in one category.

All of the above costs are then added to arrive at the cost of operation. The costs are then divided by the number of patient days to arrive at the average cost of operating the facility. An inflation factor is then applied to determine the reimbursement rate.

The real property costs are a complicated part of the formula. They are complicated for the simple reason that they are illogical, and because they are illogical, it is very difficult to explain them and have anybody make any sense out of them. It is simply the way the system is operated.

There are two rentals that we found. There is the imputed rent, and there is the maximum rent. The imputed rent is used in a non-arm's-length agreement—that is, if you owned the nursing home, and you rented it to yourself. The maximum rental is what is known as the arm's-length agreement, which is supposedly an agreement between strangers. However, according to the State Department of Health definition of a non-arm's-length agreement, if you have up to 10 percent interest in the landlord, you have a non-arm's-length agreement. That would mean, in simple terms, if your wife owned the nursing home, and rented it to you, that would be an arm's-length agreement. If your brother owned the nursing home, and rented it to you, that would be an arm's-length agreement. But what is not an arm's-length agreement is when your wife and you jointly own it—you have 50 percent and she has 50 percent—and you rent it to yourself. That is not an arm's-length agreement.

So clearly the terms "arm's-length" and "non-arm's-length" are not used in a business sense but are specialized terms. They clearly do not necessarily mean two strangers doing business together.

In New York City, where you have a lot of nursing homes that were old and were run as nursing homes for a long time, most of the rents are the maximum rental, the arm's-length agreement.

Now, for new institutions which are built, the existing rents in 1966 are used as the basis for calculating what is a fair rent.

For example, if you have an institution which contains 100 beds, and the rents, the average rents for that category of housing in New York City, or in any county of New York was $100,000, then if a new institution was built, and was on an arm's-length basis, it would also have the $100,000 maximum rental. So not merely do the 1966 rents affect those institutions which were rented in that period of time, but they affect all of the other institutions in New York, because they are used as a basis of fair comparison. Hence, we had to look very closely at what happened to those institutions, and how those rentals were calculated, and what the cost basis of those institutions were, before the Medicaid reimbursement formula started to work.

Although, the above method may appear to provide reasonable controls, there are many ways whereby fraudulent practices may enter—for instance, appointing fictitious persons to the staff and utilizing dietary and housekeeping resources for other uses.

In New York City alone, when the State Health Department auditors audit an institution, they have averaged on every institution they have audited a return of $77,000. So a $77,000 inflation factor included in here is a lot of money on each of those institutions. When we have 400 of these profitmaking institutions in New York, you have some idea of the magnitude of the moneys that are being lost by the State of New York.

One can see from the above that there is considerable room for graft, misrepresentation, and outright theft. In response to testimony like this, Congress passed P.L. 92-603, in order to focus state officials' thinking on costs and possible reduction. This law stated that as of July 1, 1976 all nursing homes were to be reimbursed on a cost-related basis. State officials were required to show how the state reimbursement levels were actually related to nursing home costs in order to receive the 50 percent federal contributions to a state's Medicaid program.

Another section of the same law stipulated that two levels of care were to be provided: the more expensive skilled nursing care and the less costly intermediate care. The difficult problem is that a decision to place persons in either level involves explicit or implicit placement assessment of the cost-related characteristics and conditions of residents.

Due to much uncertainty about the law and about the states' ability to implement the law's requirements, the law was changed. The *Federal Register* of July 1, 1976[3] clarifies the purpose, scope, and implementation of the law. Portions of this documentation follow.

Legislative Purpose of 1902(a)(13)(E)

Section 249 of Pub. L. 92-603 originated in the Senate Committee on Finance. The report of that Committee, Senate Report No. 92-1230, at pp. 287-288, indicates the legislative purposes for which section 249(a) was enacted. The Senate Report notes with concern that, without any statutory requirements that payment for medical care and services in long term care facilities be on a reasonable cost-related basis, some facilities are being overpaid by Medicaid, while others are being paid too little to support the quality of care that Medicaid patients are expected to need and receive.

The Report makes clear that the Committee was concerned about the effect of both underpayment and overpayment on the quality of medical care of recipients. If facilities are underpaid, because a State's flat rate is unrealistically low or because in determining its rate the State refuses to recognize as allowable costs some of the real costs of providing the services, facilities will be under pressure to cut corners and provide lower quality care, or will be forced to make their non-Medicaid patients absorb some of the cost of Medicaid patients' care; at worst, facilities may refuse to accept Medicaid patients. If facilities are overpaid, either because the State's flat rate is unrealistically high or because the State payment formula permits reimbursement for unnecessary items such as luxury services, questionable depreciation allowances and the like, there is little incentive for providers to employ the most efficient and economical methods of providing services, with the result that the State's Medicaid dollars do not go as far as they could to provide needed medical care. When increased inflation and unemployment are already straining State welfare budgets, this is a serious consideration. The rising costs of the Medicaid program may force a State to drop optional services or the medically needy category from its plan, as some States have already done; at worst, the high prices of medical care and services in skilled nursing facilities and intermediate care facilities might be a factor in the State's decision to drop out of the Medicaid program altogether.

Congress, then, was concerned about the harmful effects on the Medicaid program of both underpayment and overpayment of providers of long-term care facility services. On the other hand, the committee was aware that application of the reasonable cost reimbursement approach of the Medicare program to payment for long-term care facility services was not entirely satisfactory; the committee noted particularly that the tremendously detailed cost finding requirements under Medicare might be unnecessarily cumbersome and expensive.

The intent expressed in the legislative history that States be allowed the maximum possible flexibility in developing cost-related payment methods sheds light on the distinction between "reasonable cost" and "reasonable cost-related." The Senate Report declares that States need not use the Medicare reasonable cost reimbursement formula, but that they should be free to develop simpler and less expensive methodologies.

A final point on the meaning of the statutory requirement of "payment on a reasonable cost-related basis" is that the statute and the legislative history are silent on the question of the timing of such payment. The Department in these regulations makes no requirement with respect to the time of payment such as the requirement of interim payments under Medicare. Accordingly, States are free to establish such payment schedules as they find reasonable. For example, a State may wish to withhold payment or a portion of payment pending receipt of adequate cost reports from a facility. However, the Department leaves open the possibility that it may decide at some future date, on the basis of experience under these regulations, that regulatory requirements respecting the timing of payments are necessary to effectuate fully the Congressional requirement of payment on a reasonable cost-related basis.

Timetable for Implementation

A considerable number of States have expressed concern regarding the timetable for implementation of these regulations. The Department is aware that, although a good number of States will be able to implement the greater part of these regulations fairly quickly, some will need a good deal of time to begin to accumulate the cost data on which to base payment rates, and none will be able to meet all the requirements as of July 1, 1976. The Department does not intend that States should be penalized for the Department's delay in publishing final regulations. Therefore, the regulations require that the initial cost reporting period begin no later than January 1, 1977, and that States set reasonable cost-related rates no later than January 1, 1978, on the basis of cost data submitted by providers. The States are encouraged to meet each requirement of the regulations as soon as possible. Although the regulation speaks to a cost reporting period of a year, some States may set their initial rate on a cost reporting period of less than a year.

Costs of routine services: Allowable costs shall include all items of expense which providers incur in the provision of routine services. Routine services means the regular room, dietary and nursing services, minor medical and surgical supplies, and the use of equipment and facilities. Examples of expenses that allowable costs for routine services must include are:

(1) All general services including but not limited to administration of oxygen and related medications, hand-feeding, incontinency care, tray service and enemas;

(2) Items furnished routinely and relatively uniformly to all patients, such as patient gowns, water pitchers, basins and bed pans;

(3) Items stocked at nursing stations or on the floor in gross supply and distributed or used individually in small quantities; such as alcohol, applicators, cotton balls, bandaids, antacids, aspirin (and other non-legend drugs ordinarily kept on hand), suppositories, and tongue depressors;

(4) Items which are used by individual patients but which are usable and expected to be available, such as ice bags, bed rails, canes, crutches, walkers, wheelchairs, traction equipment, and other durable medical equipment;

(5) Special dietary supplements used for tube feeding or oral feeding such as elemental high nitrogen diet, even if written as a prescription item by a physician (because these supplements have been classified by the Food and Drug Administration as a food rather than a drug);

(6) Laundry services other than for personal clothing.

The ICF-SNF Differential and Supplementation Plans

The Secretary has discretion, under section 1903(h)(1) of the Act, to compute, for reimbursement purposes, a reasonable cost differential between skilled nursing facilities and intermediate care facilities.

Under this authority, the Department presently requires by regulation, at 45 CFR 250.30(b)(3)(iii)(b), that except as specified therein, to qualify for Federal financial participation the State must set its reimbursement rate for intermediate care facilities at least ten percent below the rate for skilled nursing facilities. As some comments pointed out, this differential is inconsistent with the requirement of the proposed regulations that States pay both skilled nursing and intermediate care facilities on a reasonable cost-related basis, as determined under the reimbursement principles and provisions of these regulations. In addition, a study of cost differentials between skilled nursing facilities and intermediate care facilities in five States (using cost data from 1971), conducted for the Department by a private consulting firm, indicates that there may be no rational basis for requiring any differential, since a substantial number of intermediate care facilities were found to have costs as high as those of skilled nursing facilities. The study concluded that inadequate data existed on which to base further conclusion on the question of whether any differential is appropriate.

Since section 1902(a)(13)(E) of the Act now requires that all long-term care facilities be paid on a reasonable cost-related basis, the calculation of rates in accordance with the regulation implementing this requirement should result in rates that reflect whatever differential, if any, is appropriate, without further need for a separate requirement for calculating the differential. Accordingly, the requirement for a differential has been deleted from the regulations.

In summary, if states decide to have a two-level differential of care reimbursement, they may do so. This means an assessment tool for differentiating levels of care would need to be developed. The ideal assessment tool would:

1. be based on the best possible methodology known to relate costs to characteristics.
2. have data collection costs not exceeding the benefits of assessment.
3. have explicit definitions of patient characteristics and conditions. These definitions should be able to be applied by users of different levels and different professional backgrounds.[4]

MEDICARE PROGRAM CONTROLS

The Social Security Administration is required each year to follow a federal formula in determining the future cost of the Medicare program to beneficiaries. During 1977 the nation's 25 million Medicare recipients paid a record increase in the aggregate cost of hospital and nursing home bills. Increases have been in effect on a regular basis. Moreover, as of July 1, 1977 the elderly and disabled persons receiving Medicare were paying a monthly rate of $7.70 (instead of $7.20) for medical insurance premiums. As of July 1, 1978 the rate increased to $8.20. As of July 1, 1979 it escalated to $8.70. Additional increases are surely forthcoming. The Social Security Administration indicated that the hikes were needed to keep up with skyrocketing health care costs.

During 1979 Medicare patients had to pay $160 for the first day of a hospital stay of less than 60 days. The remaining 59 days are fully covered by Medicare. The daily charge to the patient for hospitalization between 61 and 90 days amounts to $40, and after 90 days it increases to $80 per day.

In order to control the rapid increases in costs that the Social Security Administration must pay out for health care for Medicare recipients, limits on reimbursement to institutions have been introduced. It is believed a limit on reimbursement gives institutions an incentive to economize and provide more efficient care per dollar of cost.

The proposed limits and the methodology used to develop those limits follows below.[5] The limits are based on size of the SMSA (standard metropolitan statistical area) and also on other geographic location factors.

Proposed Schedule of Limits

The proposed schedule of limits on skilled nursing facility (SNF) inpatient routine service costs set forth below, when published in final, will be applicable to cost-reporting periods beginning after the effective date of the final schedule and before the effective date of a revised schedule. The proposed schedule limits will apply to the entire cost-reporting period of a skilled nursing facility whose cost-reporting period begins during the effective period of this schedule. The proposed schedule will apply to the total of the cost of routine services. These limits will not apply to the cost of ancillary services.

To permit reasonable comparison between skilled nursing facilities in a group, a classification system has been developed to take into account the economic environment of the area in which the skilled nursing facility operates. Per capita income has been used as the basis to reflect differences in input costs such as wages and costs of construction, goods, and services between various geographical areas. We have used the Standard Metropolitan Statistical Areas (SMSA) as the major geographical factor for identifying and classifying urban areas. (A Standard Metropolitan Statistical Area, as defined by the Office of Management and Budget, is a county or group of contiguous counties which (1) includes at least one city of 50,000 inhabitants, or (2) otherwise meets the basic criteria specified by the Office of Management and Budget for defining such areas. The standard definition and a complete list of SMSAs can be found in the Federal Information Processing Standards Publication (F.I.P.S. Pub.804) which is available from the Superintendent of Documents, United States Government Printing Office, Washington, D.C. 20402.) A provider location within an SMSA is used as a basis for an urban location while providers not located in an SMSA are considered nonurban.

It should be noted that bed size is not used as a classifier, as was done in setting limits on hospital inpatient general routine services because analysis of skilled nursing facility cost data indicates there is a random distribution of routine service per diem costs for small, medium, and large bed size SNFs. Because the distribution does not indicate a significant cost relationship between bed size and cost, separate limits based on bed-size categories are inappropriate in the case of SNFs. Moreover, there are no data which demonstrate that SNFs furnish significantly more complex or intensive services as they become larger in size, as is generally the case with hospitals.

Two per capita income groups are used to classify SNFs located in non-SMSA areas as compared with 5 groups used to classify hospitals in such areas. The reduction is the result of an analysis which indicates that the median routine service per diem cost of SNFs located in non-SMSA areas are so similar that they can be consolidated into 2 groups. It thus appears that the cost of providing SNF care in nonurban areas is not as sensitive to economic environment as are the costs of hospitals similarly located.

Consideration has been given to providing separate limits for hospital-based SNFs and free-standing SNFs under the rationale that the higher costs of hospital-based SNFs result because these providers have more seriously ill patients. SNF care is, by law, the next lower level of care than the care provided in a hospital and all SNFs are required to provide such care. Similarly, the Conditions of Participation and Certification Procedures are the same for all SNFs. Thus, it is reasonable to assume that all SNFs generally supply the level of care defined in regulations and that a premium reimbursement for hospital-based-SNFs merely because their costs are higher is not warranted. Any comments on this issue will be carefully evaluated in regard to the issue of whether separate limits for hospital-based SNFs are appropriate.

Methodology

To develop urban groups, the SMSAs were arrayed on the basis of their per capita income and classes were established. The nonurban groups were developed in the same manner, using per capita income of non-SMSA areas within a State. The classification system utilizes 7 classes—5 income groups for providers located in SMSA areas and 2 income groups for providers located in non-SMSA areas.

Each group list contains all the states included in the group as well as designated areas within each State. The entire list was published in the *Federal Register* of August 27, 1976.

The proposed limits were developed for each of the classification groups in the following manner:

1. Inpatient routine service cost data for each participating skilled nursing facility were obtained from the fiscal intermediaries.
2. The data for skilled nursing facilities in each class were arrayed in descending order of inpatient routine service costs.
3. The 90th percentile and median were computed for each class.
4. For each class, an amount equal to 10 percent of the median was added to the 90th percentile amount.
5. This sum was adjusted by a factor to reflect a 10 percent annual rate of estimated cost increases in per diem costs following the date of data collection.
6. The amount calculated in step 5 was rounded to the next highest dollar which establishes the limit for each class, subject to adjustment for reporting periods starting after January 1, 1976.

Under the authority of section 1861(v)(1) of the Social Security Act, it is proposed that the following cost limitations apply to the total of the skilled nursing facility inpatient routine service costs (excluding costs incurred for ancillary services), adjusted upward as provided for below. The proposed limits are applicable to cost-reporting periods beginning on or after the effective date of the final notice of these limits and will remain in effect until the effective date of a revised schedule. This schedule will apply to the entire cost-reporting period of a skilled nursing facility whose cost-reporting period begins during its effective period. Where a skilled nursing facility has a cost-reporting period beginning after January 1, 1976, the published limit will be adjusted upward by a factor of 0.833 percent for each elapsed month between January 1, 1976, and the first day of the month in which the skilled nursing facility's reporting period starts. The result of this calculation is not rounded and is to be given in dollars and cents.

Example. Skilled nursing facility A's cost-reporting period begins April 1, 1976, and ends March 31, 1977. The cost limit for skilled nursing facility A's group from the table below is $46.00.

Computation of Adjusted Cost Limit

Cost limit $46.00
Plus adjustment for 3 mo. period Jan. 1, 1976 to
Apr. 1, 1976. 3 mo. times 0.833 pct equals 2.50
pct.; 2.50 pct. times $46 .... 1.15
    Adjusted cost limit applicable to skilled nursing
    facility A for the Apr. 1, 1976 to Mar. 31,
    1977 reporting period 47.15

Schedule of Limits on Skilled Nursing Facility
Inpatient Routine Service Costs for
Skilled Nursing Facilities

Skilled Nursing Facilities Located Within SMSAs (Urban)

SMSA group:	Dollar limit
I[1]	$53
II	46
III	46
IV	37
V	43

[1]Limits apply to all Group I SMSAs except Anchorage, Alaska, and Honolulu, Hawaii, where cost-of-living adjustment was made. The limits for these areas are as follows:

Anchorage	$66
Honolulu	61

Skilled Nursing Facilities Located
Outside SMSA (Nonurban)

State group:	Dollar limit
I[2]	$47
II	40

[2]Limits apply to all group I States except Alaska and Hawaii. The limits for these areas are as follows:

Alaska	$58
Hawaii	54

CONCLUSIONS

This chapter has focused on the problems faced by lawmakers in attempting to balance two conflicting goals: quality of care and reduction of cost. Federal testimony has demonstrated how difficult it is to control the cost-reimbursement process for Medicaid. It has also been shown how Congress reacted and passed legislation to ensure that overpayment would be curbed and underpayment would be avoided—that is, to ensure that quality of care be maintained.

The similar problems faced by Medicare were also reviewed. In this case the Social Security Administration was able to increase rates to respond to Medicare expenditures. However, a reimbursement limit was set to provide an incentive for institutions to economize and provide more efficient care.

In reviewing the two reimbursement schemes by two separate federal agencies for the same types of institutional care, one wonders whether there is not a need for a more efficient and standardized federal scheme that combines two reimbursement plans under one roof. Steps toward this goal were proposed in the early months of the Carter Administration. A streamlined federal bureaucracy could result in considerable cost savings.

NOTES

1. S. Winn, "Assessment of Cost Related Characteristics and Conditions of Long Term Care Patients," *Inquiry* 12 (December 1975), p. 344–351.
2. U.S. Senate, Subcommittee on Long–Term Care of the Special Senate Committee on Aging, "Testimony on Medicaid Reimbursement Process," January 21, 1975.
3. *Federal Register* 41, no. 128 (July 1, 1976).
4. Winn, "Assessment of Cost Related Characteristics," p. 344–351.
5. *Federal Register* 41, no. 168 (August 27, 1976).

Chapter 20

Geriatric Health Manpower Development

The American medical practitioner system is organized largely along functional specialty lines. (Note that the word largely is used here to note the prominence and increasing popularity of pediatrics and the family practice specialty.) In contrast with most developed countries, the United States has so far only paid scant attention to the specialized health manpower needs of the elderly.

What is needed are geriatricians, physicians trained to respond to the special needs of the elderly. This need does not imply that senior citizens do not need the medical specialist. But the geriatrician is needed to be the primary care provider for the older person in the same way that the pediatrician is the primary care provider for the child and the family practitioner is the primary care provider for the family. Specialists will continue to be in demand for referrals in the case of specific health problems.

CURRENT STATUS OF GERIATRIC MANPOWER TRAINING

Libow[1] analyzed the reluctance of the current health care structure to provide comprehensive and/or primary care to the aged and also conducted a survey of eight United States medical schools to determine freshmen interest in obtaining specific education in geriatric medicine. Of the 629 questionnaires distributed, 52 percent were completed. The two major questions and student responses were:

1. Would you want a full course on human aging and the medical problems of the elderly?—75 percent responded *yes*
2. During your clinical years, would you want to take an elective course on the medical and psychosocial problems of the elderly?—72 percent responded *yes*

Although it appears that the majority of entering medical students are interested in having geriatric medicine and health care for the aged represented in their curriculum, the 1977–78 Association of American Medical Colleges "Curriculum Directory" shows that only 51 schools (or about 42 percent of all medical schools) offered electives in geriatrics.

Freeman[2] reported the results of a survey he conducted of the 99 United States medical schools in 1970. Eighty-five were four-year recognized schools, six were two-year basic science schools, and 8 were in a state of appraisal for four-year acceptance. Their catalogs were read to ascertain their curriculum content on aging (geriatrics, gerontology, senescence, and senility). At 51 of the 99 schools (over 50 percent), there was no mention of the subject of aging in any form in the school history, the curriculum deliberations, outline of courses, staff structure, research, or other content. Of the 48 catalogs that contained some mention of aging or gerontology, only eight specifically designated a preclinical instruction course in gerontology, and only 15 offered clinical instruction in gerontology (as a specific designation and not part of general structure). In most instances, the gerontology courses were offered in the Divisions of Psychiatry, Preventive Medicine, or Public Health. In 1970 only three schools—University of Washington, University of Chicago, and University of California at Los Angeles—had Divisions of Gerontology.

Panneton and Wesolowski[3] state that until only recently, formal education in geriatrics was extremely limited. In 1973 the American Medical Association reported that only one geriatrician was formally engaged in medical teaching. The 1978 Faculty Roster of the Association of American Medical Colleges, which includes more than forty-nine thousand paid medical school faculty edu-

Table 20-1 Summary of Geriatric Involvement by Medical Schools

	1970	1973	1978
Total number of U.S. medical schools	99		119
Total number of students enrolled			57,000
Total paid medical school faculty			49,000
Number of medical schools with Gerontology Divisions	3		
Percent of schools offering elective in gerontology			42%
Percent of schools listing a preclinical instruction course in gerontology (specifically designated and not part of another course)	8%		
Percent offering clinical instruction in gerontology (specifically designated)	15%		
Number of geriatricians employed by schools		1	
Number of faculty with primary specialization in gerontology			7
Number of faculty with secondary specialization in gerontology			13

Table 20-2 Choice of Specialty by Public Health Students

Area of Specialization	Percent of Students Choosing (n = 6,463)
Behavioral and Social Sciences	3.3
Biomedical Sciences	4.2
Biostatistics	6.8
Dental Public Health	0.9
Dietetics	0.1
Environmental Health	11.8
Epidemiology	11.8
Gerontology	*0.6*
Health Administration	16.6
Health Planning	3.4
Health Policy	2.3
Hospital Administration	4.6
International Health	2.2
Maternal and Child Health	4.1
Mental Health	2.6
Nutrition	5.9
Occupational Health	3.5
Population Studies	3.7
Public Health Education	6.5
Public Health Nursing	2.2
Public Health Social Work	0.2
Other	2.7

(Total enrollment is approximately 6,800 and includes those students who are not taking courses toward a professional degree.)

cating more than fifty-seven thousand medical students, lists only 7 faculty members with a primary specialty of geriatrics and only 13 with a secondary specialty of geriatrics. It appears, therefore, that these 20 identifiable faculty members can make little educational impact on the future physicians of this country.

Table 20-1 combines some of the pertinent information from the sources mentioned above.

Crawford[4] looked at graduate students in United States Schools of Public Health and their preferences for the various specializations offered. Professional education for public health is offered almost exclusively at the graduate level. Only 55 students were enrolled in undergraduate degree programs in 1977–78. Master's degree programs drew the bulk of public health students, with 4,839 enrolled in 1977–78. Table 20-2 indicates the percentages of students who choose the different specializations in schools of public health.

LEGISLATIVE EFFORTS TO ENCOURAGE GERIATRIC EDUCATION

Panneton and Wesolowski[5] reviewed legislative efforts to give impetus to the development of geriatric education programs. The authors point out that in the early Seventies the increase in the physician supply had been such that the Congress noted in its passage of the Health Professions Educational Assistance Act of 1976 (P.L. 94-484) that there was no longer an insufficient number of physicians and surgeons in the United States. Emphasis was now on improving the geographic and specialty distribution of health personnel.

Section 788d of P.L. 94-484 provided for training in the diagnosis, treatment, and prevention of diseases and related medical and behavioral problems of the aged. To this end, training grants for family practice and internal medicine residencies include elements of programs for the elderly. Hitherto, some 2,000 medical students and 300 faculty members have received training support in family medicine, including aspects of geriatric care.

The authors also state that the Bureau of Health Manpower's (BHM's) Division of Nursing has several provisions in the Nurse Training Act of 1975 (P.L. 94-364), that give special emphasis to the health care problems of the elderly. Six contracts, worth a total of over $2 million, were awarded in 1975 for the training of geriatric nurse practitioners. Another project under the auspices of the BHM's Division of Nursing is located in the University of Colorado Medical Center at Denver. This program prepares geriatric practitioners in long-term care facilities within a six-state area under the capitation grant program.

During 1978 representatives of the BHM, the Veterans Administration (VA), the National Institute of Aging, the American Office of Aging (AOA), the Health Care Financing Administration, the National Institute of Mental Health, and the Institute of Medicine conducted joint workshops in clinical geriatrics education. They concluded that there is a widespread need for curriculum development for health professions programs in geriatrics. Within the AOA, the new Office of Training and Education on Aging will administer a $22 million budget that stresses multidisciplinary centers. The VA has established six regional medical education centers which are to devote as much as 50 percent of their efforts to teaching geriatrics. Funds appropriated for the National Institute on Aging were increased from $34 million in 1977 to $37 million in 1978. In fiscal 1979 the appropriation was $56.9 million.

Perhaps now with these very recent efforts to enhance health care and health care education to serve the aged, the U.S. will start catching up to some of the European countries that are 10 to 20 years ahead in geriatric care. England for example, has 300 established hospital posts in geriatrics; and while England has 12 chairs in geriatrics in its medical schools, the United States has only one, es-

Table 20-3 Supply/Demand of Health Professions (in thousands)

Discipline	Supply—1980	Demand—1980	Supply—1990	Demand—1990
Physicians	444.0	425–427	594.0	543–571
Dentists	126.2	132.5	154.5	153.7
Optometrists	22.0	22.1	25.7	25.9
Podiatrists	8.7	9.9	12.5	16.1
Registered Nurses	1,152.0	1,155–1,326	1,587.0	1,571–1,885

tablished in 1977 at the Cornell Medical School. As of 1978 Russia required that geriatrics be taught in all of its 145 medical schools.

FUTURE STATUS OF HEALTH MANPOWER FOR THE AGED

In general, it is difficult to forecast the demand for any type of health professionals, and this extends as well to geriatric-related health practitioners. Furthermore, as expressed by Stambler,[6] no current method of predicting future requirements is without significant conceptual data and problems; different analytical approaches often provide different end results. Stambler reports on the results of a study by the Bureau of Health Manpower/Manpower Analysis Branch,[7] and, in further delineating the limitations of manpower projections, states that factors such as shortages or surpluses of physicians' services either by specialty, setting, or geographic location that exist in the current system are usually carried through the projections. However, basic changes in the system such as instituting national health insurance or hospital cost controls are not incorporated. The BHM study[8] provided the data shown in summary form in Table 20-3. The ranges given for the need for both physicians and registered nurses in the years 1980 and 1990 reflect the different models currently being evaluated by the BHM.

OBSTACLES TO DEVELOPMENT OF GERIATRIC HEALTH MANPOWER

Although the health manpower projections are a reasonably good indication of the supply and demand for health practitioners in the years given, their direct relationship to meeting the health needs of the elderly is absent. For this, turn to the testimony of Dr. Leslie Libow.[9] Libow is the chairman of the Clinical Section Gerontological Society and Director of the Long Island Jewish Institute for Geriatric Care. He reported in May 1978 to the House Select Committee on Aging on the need for geriatricians (physicians who specilize in geriatric care).

Libow stated that there is a current need for a cadre of eight to ten thousand geriatricians. This need represents 3.3 percent of the total number of physicians now in practice. The cadre was broken down into disciplines and included nearly five hundred located in medical schools, seven thousand in skilled nursing facilities, and twenty-four hundred in training hospitals.

With such impressive utilization rates of health care services in this country, why have the health care problems of the elderly not been approached more vigorously? Libow cited the following reasons:[10]

- *Ageism*—This is defined as an inherent prejudice against the elderly. Central to this concept is the widespread fear of growing old. Physicians feel this fear as strongly as everyone else. This fear often leads to a denial of the existence of the elderly and/or their special problems.

- *Professional territoriality*—If a new area of geriatric medicine were to develop, internists, family practitioners, neurologists, psychiatrists, and other health professionals would tend to be unnecessarily apprehensive about their competition and the boundaries of their competitors.

- *Patient passivity*—The aged themselves have not vigorously demanded improvements in meeting their health care needs.

- *Time-income factor*—The earning power of the primary care physician is closely related to the number of patients seen per unit of time. Thus, the elderly, who often display multiple problems and require more time for proper evaluation, are viewed as a losing proposition.

- *Educators' attitudes*—Medical educators frequently—and inaccurately— believe that the training of students and resident physicians in geriatric care is already done at other schools. However, this responsibility is claimed by very few schools. As stated by Libow, "the teaching of the special psychosocial, biologic, and medical aspects of growing old needs more emphasis in medical school, residency, and continuing medical education programs."

- *Medicare*—While Medicare's increased payments to practitioners and institutions have brought better and more treatment to the ailing organs of the elderly, Medicare has not brought an improvement in primary care. In fact, Medicare can be viewed as an obstacle to the development of an overall health care system for the aged, including such facets as preventive health care and health education. Each agent of the health care system now attempts to render maximum treatment to a specific problem or defective organ, exhausting the limited money, time, and energy that could be used instead to provide the elderly with comprehensive, coordinated health care.

CONCLUSIONS

Whereas geriatrics is a common profession in most developed countries, it is not so in the United States. Not only is there a paucity of geriatrician training programs in American medical schools, there is also little interest in gerontology in United States Schools of Public Health.

Although nursing is not as specialized as most other health professions, there appears to be little interest in geriatric training. The training of geriatric nurse practitioners is also in its initial state.

NOTES

1. L. Libow, "The Issues in Geriatric Medical Education," *Geriatrics* (February 1977): 99–102.

2. J. T. Freeman, "A Survey of Geriatric Education—Catalogues of U.S. Medical Schools," *Journal of the American Geriatric Society* 19 (September 1971): 746–62.

3. P. E. Panneton and E. F. Wesolowski, "Current and Future Needs in Geriatric Education," *Public Health Reports* 94 (January-February 1979): 73–79.

4. B. L. Crawford, "Graduate Students in U.S. Schools of Public Health," *Public Health Reports* 94 (January-February 1979): 67–72.

5. Panneton and Wesolowski, "Current and Future Needs," p. 73–79.

6. H. V. Stambler, "Health Manpower for the Nation—A Look Ahead at the Supply and the Requirements," *Public Health Reports* 94 (January-February 1979): 3–10.

7. Manpower Analysis Branch, Bureau of Health Manpower, Health Resources Administration: *A Report to the President and Congress on the Status of Health Professions Personnel in the U.S.*, DHEW Publication–HRA-78-93 (Washington, D.C.: U.S Government Printing Office, 1978).

8. Ibid.

9. U.S. Congress, Select Committee on Aging (Washington, D.C.: U.S. Government Printing Office, May 17, 1978).

10. Libow, "The Issues in Geriatric Medical Education," p. 99–102.

Chapter 21

Terminal Care—Issues and Alternatives[*]

In this chapter the authors, Claire F. Ryder and Diane M. Ross, delve into the problematic issues associated with caring for terminally ill patients. Traditionally, terminally ill persons die in an institutional setting. What is proposed is to transfer them to a home or homelike environment where they would be able to share their last moments with relatives in a pleasant environment.

Of course, the objective of the medical profession and the hospital is to cure and rehabilitate patients. Cure and rehabilitation are measures of success. Caring for patients afflicted with degenerative diseases is a task that runs counter to the interests of the typical health care provider.

Claire F. Ryder, MD, MPH, is Director, Division of Policy Development, Office of Long Term Care, Public Health Service. Diane Ross, BA, is currently working toward a MPH degree at the University of California at Los Angeles.

As the aim of contemporary medicine moves more clearly to diagnosis and cure, the criterion of rehabilitation potential has been a deciding factor for reimbursable services under Title XVIII of the Social Security Act. However, with the increasing ability of medical technology to prolong life past its natural point, with slight chance of recovery, the prevailing criterion has been questioned. The definition of skilled care in skilled nursing facilities, as published in the September 24, 1975, *Federal Register* is that:

> The restoration potential of a patient is not the deciding factor in determining whether a service is to be considered skilled or non-

---

[*] This chapter originally appeared as an article by Claire F. Ryder and Diane M. Ross in *Public Health Reports* 92, no. 1 (January-February 1977): 20–29. It is reprinted with permission.

skilled. Even where full recovery or medical improvement is not possible, skilled care may be needed to prevent, to the extent possible, deterioration of the condition or to sustain current capabilities. For example, even though no potential for rehabilitation exists, a terminal cancer patient may require skilled services as defined . . .

Such emphasis is characteristic of an increasing interest in death and dying, by the public as well as health professionals, that has triggered greater attention to the care of the terminally ill generally and the needs of individual dying patients and their families. These needs, ranging from relief of physical pain to emotional support, require services that are not readily met in a conventional hospital or skilled nursing facility. Because the aim of treatment is "to preserve life and to relieve distress, to palliate, to maintain comfortable existence as long as possible,"[1] many health professionals have proposed removing terminal patients from a traditional institutional setting. Consequently, these professionals have attempted to create programs in home care and in inpatient facilities specifically geared for terminal patients and their families. These innovations will require a change in Federal policy, and, in fact, will demand long-term legislative change, which, in turn, must take into account:

1. The attitude of community leadership, health professionals, and the public to deny the reality of death and needs of the patient and family.
2. Inadequate services to meet the needs of the patient and family.
3. Inadequate financing mechanisms.
4. Inadequate information regarding cost effectiveness of alternatives to traditional institutional care for the terminally ill patient.

OUR CHANGING SOCIETY

Basic to our failures in the care of "the terminally ill is the fact that American society in its preoccupation with perpetual youth, beauty, sexuality, and strength has typically disguised, avoided, denied and embellished death" resulting in alienation of the dying.[2a] This isolation has been encouraged by a change in societal institutions, most prevalent of which is the change in family structure, a metamorphosis that followed economic evolution from the extended family to the modern nuclear family. Within the extended family, the processes of the life cycle were an accepted and natural part of daily life, with birth and death on a continuum in nature. Ill persons were cared for in their homes by their families, and the burials of those who died were attended by all members of the family.

With the emergence of industrialization and urbanization, the family ceased to function as the sole support of the individual, resulting in mobility and a schism between occupation and home. The extended family was whittled down as the middle-class young gravitated toward the suburbs and left the old and the poor isolated in urban centers. With the aging thus removed from the nuclear family, the succeeding generations became desensitized to death of the old. In addition, the establishment of hospitals isolated the ill. Therefore, because people rarely saw death, they could avoid it and in doing so, feared it.[2b]

Concurrent with technological changes that altered the family structure were those that altered morbidity and mortality rates. From 1900 to the present, the life expectancy at birth has increased substantially, from 47 to 70 years. However, along with changes in overall death rates came changes in causes of death. Infant and maternal mortality rates have sharply declined, and infectious diseases have been replaced by heart disease and cancer as leading causes (67 percent) of U.S. deaths. Concomitantly, these degenerative diseases are classified as long-term or terminal illness in that the prognosis given indicates a time limit on a person's survival. Thus, a new problem in the health field is the care of persons with lingering illnesses.[3]

PROFESSIONAL ATTITUDES TOWARD DEATH AND DYING

The present orientation of the medical profession is not in caring for patients afflicted with degenerative diseases but in curing them. Technological breakthroughs in medicine have perpetuated a phenomenon found among health professionals as well as in the society at large, a phenomenon referred to as "death denying." Until recently, this attitude was reflected in the training of physicians and nurses. Recurrent in the medical student's education was the idea that "every death corresponds to a failure, either of the individual physician, or more commonly, of medicine, as a whole:"[4a] The student becomes desensitized to death symbols—blood, bone, corpses, and the characteristic stench—and through transference may become desensitized to death itself.[4b] In his dedication to the ideals of the scientific community, the physician responds with "vigorous application of laboratory diagnostic tests, technological gadgetry, and heroic therapy in order to prolong life."[4c] Therefore, whereas 50 years ago the physician was considered a member of a consolatory profession, science has now given him omnipotent powers to keep the vital functions of a body operative by artificial means long after the natural course of disease has vitiated these functions.

Thus, the new orientation of physicians reduces the crux of the problem to the question: When does death occur? Much of the current literature deals with ethical and legal questions surrounding the point of death and delineates problems that occur when the prolongation of life past its natural point preempts death as a natural process. We are now at the point where considerations of quality of life are secondary to concern about the length of life. Quality of life is a subjective assessment, but when applied to the terminal patient as primary to the length of survival, it takes on specific meaning. One can debate whether survival amid tubes and respirators is life at all.

WHERE PEOPLE DIE

As mentioned previously, the home no longer provides a person with an extensive support system. In light of this, it is not surprising that the death rate in institutions has risen considerably over the past decades. Although national statistical studies pertaining to deaths in institutions as opposed to deaths at home are scarce, some State and local data are available. From 1949 to 1958, a 10 percent national increase occurred in institutional deaths, including those in general hospitals, mental hospitals, and nursing homes. New York statistics reveal an increase from 53,746 institutional deaths in 1955 to 64,083 in 1967, representing a 7 percent increase, and a 7 percent decrease in deaths at home, from 25,598 in 1955 to 21,222 in 1967.[3] Furthermore, there is evidence that this latter figure has decreased rapidly in more recent years.

Paradoxically, a survey of deaths from cancer between 1969 and 1971 in south-central Connecticut showed that 67 percent of these patients had expressed a desire to die at home as opposed to the 20 percent who did die at home. In addition, this study revealed a significant difference from a socioeconomic point of view. Those in the upper socioeconomic level were more successful in meeting their desires as were many in the low socioeconomic group, although for disparate reasons. The upper income group had the advantage of personal control, private health insurance, and monetary resources to aid in keeping the patient home. However, the low socioeconomic group and lower-middle class were successful because of reimbursement for care services under Medicaid, as well as support supplied by a cohesive extensive family. The report of this survey, prepared for the National Cancer Institute, identifies the upper-middle class as unique:

> In the upper-middle class, the resources of Medicaid are not available and Medicare is only available for patients over 65. It should also be noted that visiting nurses are most effective in a family situation where there are several primary care givers to relieve one another from the emotional and physical burdens of the care. In the upper-middle class family, it is our observation that when the family care giver is a man, he usually keeps on working, ergo the necessity for

some form of institutionalization where the upper-middle class has better insurance coverage.

Since 70 percent of institutionalization for the terminally ill pertains to the general hospital, the burden of care is placed largely on the hospital staff.[5] However, the organizational structure of the hospital makes care routinized rather than individualized, and is, therefore, frequently inappropriate to the needs of the dying patient. The large teaching hospital's primary functions are diagnosis and treatment of patients with acute illnesses. In contrast, the chronic illness hospital or wing, which houses a large population of dying patients, is generally relegated a lowersocial status, and thereby has difficulty in attracting funding and quality staff. The hierarchy for patient care in a general hospital is (*a*) acute illness, (*b*) chronic illness, and (*c*) terminal illness.[6]

The medical staff adheres to this hierarchy in its orientation toward care. As more demands of physical care of those with acute curable illnesses are met, the psychological and emotional needs of the incurable are more often neglected. Physicians tend to view cure as their triumph and death as their failure; they therefore attend to dying patients as prescribed only by duty. Nurses tend to "pull away" from dying patients and to focus more on the diagnostic and curative aspects that are implicit in their trained professional approach to patients.[7] According to Sheldon and associates:[8]

... conceptual limitations include an inability to perceive and interact with the psychological and social needs of patients and their families, a lack of effective communication among physicians, nurses, and other ward personnel, and a failure to appreciate the emotional and psychological difficulties that characterize the medical staff's reaction to patient problems.

Patients suffering from cancer are often shuttled from one specialist to another, which results in further fragmentation of care rather than an integration of services encompassing the physical, social, and emotional needs of the patient.

Pain is singularized as physiological pain that can be easily treated with the use of psychopharmacological agents. These agents often replace staff contact, which, in the case of the dying patient, is already minimized. The psychological experience of the patient and family "is deadened by the use of narcotic and analgesic drugs which reinforce the collusion of avoidance rather than enhance the experience of death."[9] The drugs aid in meeting the goal of patient manageability, essential in a busy hospital.

Terminal patients also die in nursing or convalescent homes, many of which are classified as skilled nursing facilities. These facilities are often not oriented to meet the needs of the dying patient, focusing on physical rehabilitation or restoration rather than on the total needs of the patient. In a 1975 survey of 77 nursing homes,[10] a majority indicated that they removed deceased patients as clandestinely as possible so as not to disturb the other residents—a practice that seeks to deny death by making it a covert issue.

SOCIAL DEATH VERSUS BIOLOGICAL DEATH

The result of the institutionalization of dying patients is a phenomenon of "social death" prior to biological death, which incorporates "the process of mutual disengagement and rejection by which 'organization man'—more precisely, the human being as a member of society—seems prone to take his leave from the land of the living."[11a] Once the patient has been labeled terminal and the physician has given up hope for recovery, the institution treats the patient as a dying body with little concern for his individuality or humanness. Sudnow[11b] in his study of a county hospital, observed:

> When a physician abandons hope for a patient's survival, the nurses establish what they refer to as a "death watch," a fairly severe form of social death in which they keep track of relevant facts concerning the gradual recession of clinical life signs. As death approaches, the patient's status as a body becomes more evident from the manner in which he is discussed, treated, and moved about. Attention shifts from concern about his life, possible discomforts, and the administration of medically prescribed treatments to the mere activity of the events of biological leave-taking.
>
> In a patient who has not yet passed into a death coma, suctioning the nasal passages, propping up pillows, changing bed sheets, and the like occur as part of the normal nursing routine. As blood pressure drops, and signs of imminent death appear, these traditional nursing practices are regarded as less important, the major items of interest become the number of heartbeats and changing condition of the eyes. On many occasions nurses' aides in the county hospital were observed to cease administering oral medications when death was expected within the hour.

When social death precedes biological death in this manner, the needs of the dying patient essentially become secondary to institutional routine. What are these unique needs and how are they met? Hospice, Inc., New Haven, Conn., in a study of cancer deaths between 1969 and 1971 in the South Central Health Planning Region in Connecticut summarized these needs:[5]

(1) the noxious symptoms of the illness, (2) the need to be with family and friends in familiar surroundings, (3) involvement in decision-making, (4) honest and frequent communication, (5) a need to maintain one's identity and role, (6) freedom from heroic measures which become more of an obstacle to the quality of life than even the disease, (7) need for a staff which understands and helps the patient work through anger and depression in coming to terms with dying, and (8) unattended bereavement which results in physical and/or psychological impairment to the survivors.

In a 1975 symposium on the terminally ill, Dr. Balfour Mount, medical director of the Royal Victoria Hospital's terminal patient ward in Montreal, Canada, noted that each need is interconnected and that all needs essentially signify relief from pain. Although all else is secondary to physical pain and must be dealt with before any other consideration, a hospital environment often limits the definition of pain to somatic. An expanded definition would include mental, financial, interpersonal, and spiritual aspects of pain. The dying patient may experience a sense of isolation, especially in a hospital setting, because of a lack of comfort and communication with medical personnel and family. Physicians, in avoiding the reality of death and projecting their fears onto the patient, often choose not to disclose the prognosis of impending death to the patient. Hence, an aura of deceit and covertness hampers the patient's ability to cope with his situation and to take care of unfinished business.

COPING WITH DYING AND DEATH

The coping process involves several stages, the transition from one to another being facilitated by a neutral uninvolved party, be it physician, nurse, social worker, professional counselor, member of the clergy, or understanding volunteer. The stages, as outlined by Ross,[12] are (a) denial, (b) anger, (c) bargaining, and (d) acceptance, each with its unique reactions and communication patterns. The patient experiences these various emotions in regard to his finiteness, successes, failures, family, all tied together into a package of fear, guilt, and an intense desire, on the part of many, to remain independent. The concerns of dying patients, of course, vary with age—the young girl feeling alienated from companions, the mother worried about the burden of her family and the safety of her children, the successful businessman concerned about his finances—all essentially emphasizing the need to retain a unique identity. This realization of individuality is in conflict with the treatment of only the physical discomfort of the deteriorating body rather than the whole human being with a past and a present.

The mental anguish of a person approaching death is intrinsically bound to interpersonal communication with those who are close to him, usually the family. In actuality, the needs of the family are so closely interwoven with the patient's needs, that to deny the former is to hinder the patient's process of acceptance. Indeed, often the family must experience the same mental stages as the patient's. Communication is enhanced by a realistic, honest expression of feeling through which both the patient and family are relieved of guilt. Often a "game" is played between spouses that consists of hiding knowledge of impending death from each other. Until both parties can communicate and share this knowledge progress toward mutual acceptance of the inevitable is halted. Again, each patient and family unit's problems and the manner in which they are most appropriately handled are unique.

Financial considerations are an undeniable aspect of the problems of coping with terminal illness. According to a Department of Health, Education and Welfare Report of the Task Force on Medicaid and Related Programs (cited by Pollack[13]), "the catastrophically ill are at almost any income level where insurance benefits (including the most liberal major medical coverage) do not cover the cost of sustaining expensive, long-term illnesses." Generally, those under 65 years of age are not eligible for Medicare and those above a certain income level (specified by each State) are not covered by Medicaid. A study by Cancer Care, Inc., in 1973,[14] revealed that the median cost incurred by the families of cancer patients was $19,055 which is two and two-thirds times more than the median family income of $8,000. Such universal inability to meet the high cost of hospitalization, surgery, and other treatment strikes hard at the nerve of the patient's guilt, as he may feel personally responsible for the foregone education of a child or the general depletion of the family funds for the future. Financial difficulties may trigger maladjustments as family members may be forced to adopt new roles; for example, housewife turned sole supporter.

Of course, the spiritual needs of a patient are an individual matter. Each person copes with religion or the absence or religion in his own way. Although some attempt to deal with death as the cessation of existence of the mind and body, many patients need to view their death in a religious context, either in relation to a deity or to nature, or both. There are as many perceptions of death as there are people, including concepts such as an indestructible soul, continuation with nature, reunion with Christ, or continuity through survivors. Each patient should be encouraged to express his feelings about death.

The ultimate culmination of a dying person's needs is dignity of personhood in living and in death. It may be argued as to the definition of "death with dignity," some attesting that this implies accepting death, others claiming that this infers dying in the fashion in which one lived; for example, a hostile person would die with the grudge he carried with him through life. Nevertheless, the crux of dying with dignity is in retaining one's individuality, be that in acceptance or denial, anger or serenity, without the humiliation of unnecessary life-prolonging machines.

Although the concerns of the patient cease with the end of his life, the problems of the family linger; in fact, they often intensify with the patient's death. The length and pattern of bereavement is contingent upon the relationship of the survivor to the deceased and the degree to which communication channels were open during the dying process of the patient, relating to identification with the patient, working through ambivalent feelings, and the satisfaction of mutual dependency needs.[15] Hospital environments seldom are conducive to laying the groundwork for a normal bereavement period as relatives are rushed in and out at prescribed visiting hours, children are not allowed to visit patients, and there are incidents of the family being pushed into the hallways while the patient is pronounced dead by a hurried physician who is not capable of dealing with the emotional reaction of the family.

THE HOSPICE CONCEPT

In attempts to deal with all these very special needs of the dying patient and his family, various plans in the United States and Canada have adopted the paradigm of caring for the total patient and family needs with the ideals set forth in the hospice concept. This concept is used in two British facilities which serve as prototypes. Saunders,[16] medical director of the largest of these models, St. Christopher's Hospice in London, speaks of the goals of this concept as individualization of death and relief of distress:

> The name hospice, "a resting place for travellers or pilgrims," was chosen because this will be something between a hospital and a home, with the skills of the one and the hospitality, warmth, and the time available of the other and beds without invisible parking meters beside them. We aim, above all, to recognise the interest and importance of the individual who must be helped to live until he dies and who, as he does so in his own way, will find his "own" death with quietness and acceptance. A staff who recognise this as their criterion of success will not find this work negative or discouraging and will know that it is important, both in its own right and also in all the implications it holds for the rest of medicine and, indeed, the rest of life.

St. Christopher's Hospice is a 54-bed inpatient facility for people who are in the advanced stages of neurological and malignant diseases. The foremost concern is the relief of the symptoms that often become so closely interwoven with mental anguish. Common problems in addition to pain are nausea and vomiting, constipation, diarrhea, anorexia, and anticholinergic effects. It is essential that the patient be as symptom free as possible, so that the dying does not derive from the symptoms rather than the disease. Tension and anxiety can result from the common practice of withholding medication until the pain has become incapacitating. Furthermore, this may cause the patient to become dependent, not only on the drug but on the person who administers it. St. Christopher's Hospice makes a practice of giving a fixed dosage continually in anticipation of the pain so that the patient never knows the severe potential of the pain. A common pain killer used for this purpose is Bromtom's mixture, a concoction of heroin, cocaine, alcohol, and fruit syrup—understandably, the possibility of addiction is not of concern. In addition, steroids are used to enhance the sense of well-being, to improve the appetite, to relieve pain and lower the narcotic dose, to reduce inflammation, and to alleviate weakness. In short, great care is given to the relief of pain and, in turn, to relieve mental anguish and to facilitate awareness of the experience of living until death.

The importance of living until death as a positive fulfillment necessitates an interdisciplinary staff. Each aspect of care is essential to meet the goal of total patient and family unit, including physical, mental, interpersonal, and spiritual elements. As the primary evaluator and prescriber of a medication regimen, the physician is an essential member of the hospice team. His concern for the patient's mental and physical comfort moves him to open channels of communication. As Cotter observes:[17]

> In ways unique to the relationship with each individual patient, caring enables the doctor to discern the patient's desire to discuss the future course of his illness, the nearness of his death, and the circumstances which may surround it, as well as the ways in which his family may best be supported in bearing this knowledge.

This sharing allows both the patient and family to discuss matters openly and permits them to "say goodbye," which studies have revealed as important. The physician is essentially in an omnipotent position to help this exchange or to "inflict wounds by his own thoughtlessness or need to hurry away from something that is very hard to witness."[18]

In the hospice, the nursing staff must be sensitive to the elements of human dignity. They must be aware of individual differences and responses in personal care because many patients have become quite helpless, and the nurses must convey feelings of compassion and understanding for the person's integrity and retention of uniqueness. The nurses must relay any changes in the patient's condition to the physician, so that appropriate adjustments may be made in medication as well as to the patient's daily needs for food and fluid intake, oral hygiene, and body positioning. Cotter points this out:[17]

> Taking time to explain procedures, to honor preferences, to respect privacy and modesty, to consult with the patient concerning his feelings and his needs, to involve him in social and recreational activities and in small celebrations reflect the nurse's recognition of the patient's personal worth and convey to him the certainty that he still matters, that he has not been "written off" as finished.

The emphasis on religion in this therapeutic community takes on a new meaning of the spiritual. At St. Christopher's, a church-based institution, there is an involvement of clergy and other church-based personnel whose vocation is founded in such work. However, there is an active application of McMurray's definition of religion that "it is the field of personal relationships between people prepared to give themselves to each other in the context of a common life."[19a] The religious commitment of St. Christopher's is thus manifested in its very existence as a community of vulnerable, caring, and involved people, including professionals, volunteers, patients, families, and visitors.

Although substantial attention is given to inpatient care within the physical structure of St. Christopher's, where 400 patients die each year, 10 to 15 percent of the patients are discharged home for a period of time before death. The staff realizes the value of home care by allowing the patient to feel a part of his family and to return to a relative degree of normalcy, however limited and temporary.

In essence, St. Christopher's Hospice has successfully combined the art of medicine with its value and judgment, with the science of medicine to assuage the pains of patients as they approach death, and with help for their families. The prevailing ideology is succinctly summed up in Saunders' assessment:[19b] "There is a stage when the treatment of a hemorrhage is not another transfusion; but adequate sedation, or someone who will not go away but will stay and hold a hand."

AN AMERICAN MODEL

In an attempt to fill the existing gap in the health care system regarding services for the terminally ill, various facilities and organizations have incorporated the ideals of St. Christopher's Hospice. The most successful U.S. model to date is Hospice, Inc., of New Haven, Conn. Under a National Cancer Institute grant, a 44-bed inpatient facility for cancer patients is being planned. Using St. Christopher's Hospice as a model, Hospice, Inc., services are meant to:[5]

(1) provide medical care for the continuing control of symptoms such as pain, nausea, anorexia, etc.; (2) concentrate on bedside nursing to provide comfort, close attention to easing physical distress, slow lengthy encounters that allow for the patient's care, interpersonal interactions, attention to feeding, emotional support, etc.; (3) focus on the family unit and allow the patient and family to use the assets of their life-style to cope with the situation; (4) include the patient and family by being very careful to develop good open communications; (5) involve the community by including volunteers, many of whom are widows or widowers, in varied activities from assisting with patient care to gardening, assisting in the day-care center, helping in the business office; (6) provide spiritual care through ecumenical services, discussion groups, and through an atmosphere of love and concern; (7) include an outpatient and inpatient program to provide a comprehensive program to meet different patient/family needs; (8) have a carefully constructed facility which fosters a spirit of friendliness, encourages individuals to participate in life, and is more homelike than hospitals; and (9) have built-in supports for staff and volunteers so that they can carry on demanding work.

Since March 1974, Hospice has serviced 85 families through its home care program, guided by the philosophy that, it is hoped, will continue through completion of the inpatient facility—that the patient should be maintained in the home as long as possible before being institutionalized. The program is under the medical direction of Dr. Sylvia Lack, who heads a staff consisting of two part-time physicians, six registered nurses, two licensed practical nurses, a social worker, a director of volunteers, and an admissions registrar. Consultant staff includes a clinical pharmacologist, a psychiatrist, a radiologist, and a physical therapist. In addition, there are 50 volunteers who had been carefully screened and given extensive orientation before they were assigned to specific patients. The home care program is coordinated with hospitals in the vicinity and includes medical and nursing consultation and family counseling and pain consultation and services on a 24-hours-a-day basis. All staff members are available on call, through an answering and paging service—an essential element, not only for complete service but for the confidence of the patient and family unit of care. Eligibility for participation requires residence within a specific geographic area and is contingent upon a referral from a primary care physician who is involved throughout the duration of the patient's illness.

The success of Hospice, Inc., has established the program as a national demonstration center and has encouraged other medical and nursing personnel to investigate possibilities for establishment of similar programs, in their respective geographic locations. One such program operates under the title Hospice of

Santa Barbara, Inc., a nonprofit voluntary agency incorporated in December 1974. Since September 1975, it has been operating as an information and referral service for those terminal patients and their families who suffer from uncontrolled pain of a physical, psychological, social, or spiritual nature. No special plans have been made as yet regarding an inpatient facility, because the present focus is on the home care program, which started on a pilot basis on December 1, 1975. The program was certified as a home health agency with contracts with two visiting nurse associations for the provision of skilled nursing care. The personnel of Hospice of Santa Barbara include a medical social worker, a part-time physician, a part-time pharmacist, a medical records librarian, and an executive director.

OTHER CARE PROGRAMS

This emphasis on home care must not be underplayed. Studies have revealed that people prefer to die at home or, at least, remain at home for as long as possible, for they often feel lonely and isolated within a sterile institutional setting. Within this framework, an increasing number of institutions, which do not care for the terminal patient within the facility for monetary or other reasons, nevertheless do provide home care services. In addition to being psychologically preferred by many patients, it appears from informal statements that the cost factor for home care is well below that of hospitalization. For example, Dr. Balfour Mount, at the symposium mentioned earlier, claimed that his hospital's home care program saves the equivalent of $100,000 per year as compared to the cost of hospitalization. Jack Lally of the Cardinal Ritter Institute of St. Louis, Mo., a home health agency, cited the following comparative figures based on the actual cost of home care for 140 terminally ill patients for about 4 months in contrast to what the cost would have been for varying patterns of care for that same period in 1972:

Source of care	*Cost*
Home	$ 94,000
Hospital	1,768,000
Nursing home	350,000
Home and last 2 weeks in hospital	162,000

Although it is apparent that home care is both economically and psychologically feasible, it is not adequate by itself—rather, it is most effective when used in conjunction with some type of facility, be it hospital, nursing home, or hospice. There often comes a point when a family is no longer able to keep the patient at home for medical or emotional reasons. In fact, there is often an interplay throughout the illness between institutional and home care. This shuffle between hospital, home, and nursing home poses a problem in reimbursement policies under Medicare in that admission to a skilled nursing facility after a prolonged stay at home must be preceded by a 3-day hospital stay before reimbursement can be made.

As the movement for hospices has grown, many institutions have incorporated the ideals set forth by St. Christopher's Hospice within a conventional hospital setting, as a separate ward for the terminally ill. Lamerton cites Saunders' support for a separate unit of care:[20]

> A unit for patients with advanced or terminal cancer does not have the challenge of diagnosis nor difficult decisions to make concerning radical treatment. It does not have the interest and encouragement of cure and only rarely of remission, but it is easier for its workers to look at their patients as people, to spend time with their relatives and concentrate on the relief of distress whenever it appears. Above all, it should be easier for them to give a patient the kind of unhurried attention he needs so greatly.

This is the philosophy behind the Life Acceptance Program in the Pinecrest Hospital of Santa Barbara, Calif. Within this unit, which has a fairly rapid turnover, there are from 6 to 12 patients at any one time. Two problems exist: (a) because of staffing needs and other undefined logistical reasons, the unit is required to include stroke rehabilitation; this presents a conflict since the rehabilitative needs of the stroke patient are quite divergent from the needs of terminal patients who have no rehabilitative potential and (b) frequently, physicians do not assess patients as terminally ill until they are semicomatose, thus giving the staff a brief and inadequate 48 to 72 hours to get to know a patient and his family. Because such care for patient and family is not begun until the patient is transferred to this special ward, fragmented care results.

A strong argument is made by Lamerton against the isolation of the dying in a general hospital:[20]

> I do not see a special terminal ward within a general hospital as a good solution, either. Those nurses who did not want to do this kind of work would dread being posted to the ward and would not be the right people to work in it. Matron (or do I mean the chief, principal senior, or nursing officer?) would be overheard to say, "I can't help it, we have three nurses off sick in the acute surgical ward; they'll just have to be brought from the Dead End." Consequently, the terminal unit would be permanently understaffed.

Another case is made against the segregation of the terminally ill in the philosophy and practice of Veterans Administration programs for these patients.

Their policy is that such isolation is highly detrimental since the patient is thus labeled as dying or "hopeless." Others have verbalized this objection, which appears to be valid when viewed within the context of a society that has not, on the whole, considered death a natural process. With this in mind, indeed such labeling can be deleterious.

Thus, the third alternative to employing the hospice concept is the hospital that does not segregate its terminally ill, but caters to their special needs. One such plan is used at the Harrisburg (Pa.) Hospital, a 450-bed general hospital, where the success is attributed to one nurse, Joy Ufema. She dubbed the "death and dying specialist," claims that the hospice concept is more dependent on an administrative commitment than on an edifice. Working as the patient's advocate, she has developed the skill of listening, allowing the patient to make his own decisions by asking: What do you need? Whom do you need? When do you need it? She then proceeds to satisfy these needs, with the help of a very cooperative social service department and the patient's family.

The Harrisburg model is used by hospitals that have some plans for a terminal unit, but for financial and logistical reasons, the plans remain long range. There are indications that some members of hospital staffs, often a member of the clergy, are attempting to attend to dying patients in a unique way. Rev. Leroy Joesten, pastoral care director of Lutheran General Hospital, Park Ridge, Ill., in a personal communication, described the staff's orientation:

> It is important to say that our hospital's approach to care of the dying is to deal with it in the total context of care and treatment of a disease. Hence, each of our medical and surgical units functions from a multidisciplinary model directed at "total patient care." This total care attempts to address terminal care needs for patients, family, and staff as well as curative and palliative care needs.

The key to this type of care is a commitment by the entire staff— administration, medical, nursing, and social service. However, the feasibility within the framework of a general hospital is dubious because, as previously discussed, hospitals are routinized for the purpose of curing the acutely ill. Catering to dying patients' needs is often at the risk of disrupting patterns that, perhaps, were created for efficient and effective treatment of those with rehabilitative potential. The individual needs of terminal patients seemed to be best tended outside such an environment.

COST FACTOR

The case for the viability of a hospice as a freestanding facility can be argued on two fronts: (*a*) care effectiveness and (*b*) cost effectiveness. Thus far, most of the literature has dealt with the effective care factor. It has been shown that the present orientation of medical personnel, hospitals, and nursing homes, as it exists today, is incompatible with hospice ideals. The cost factor has only been estimated without the aid of a formalized study. Lack[21] projects a cost of $105 a day in New Haven for a hospice room in 1977–78, the planned completion date for the inpatient facility. This figure should be compared with an estimated $190 a day in a general hospital in that vicinity, at that projected time. The cost differential is attributed to a hospital's overhead costs due to "the operating rooms, the specialized care areas, the machines for extending life beyond its natural term."[21] Although services that are integral to patient assessment and treatment will be included, such as a pharmacy with a full-time pharmacist to provide the pain-control medication needs, diagnostic radiology, oxygen, suction systems available at every bed, and a small laboratory to conduct the most frequently administered testing procedures, Hospice, Inc., of New Haven will rely on neighboring hospitals for services such as chemotherapy, palliative radiation therapy, and surgical units, if necessary.

The cost factor also includes the price of erecting special structures. Hospice's 1975 annual report quotes $1,325,000 for planning and building the facility. The consideration to be made is whether the amount saved over general hospitalization costs merits the high cost of building new facilities when there is a plethora of beds in existing community hospitals. In a 1975 lecture in Brantford, Conn., Mount cited a possible impracticality in reference to St. Christopher's Hospice, which serves 54 patients within a 6-mile radius: "This does not encompass even half the target population and leaves 70 percent of the patients in need dying in institutions." Thus, the incurred cost of building hospices may benefit only a minority of those in need, while simultaneously diverting attention from demands that need to be met within hospitals.

SUMMARY AND CONCLUSION

The most desired goal for patients and concerned health professionals is home care for the terminally ill. The familiar surroundings and faces help to relieve the psychological suffering encountered in the dying process and allow freer communication channels between patient and family. However, it is apparent that during some point in the last weeks of life the patient may require closer medical supervision for pain relief, or the family may not be able to continue care once the patient has reached a certain phase, thereby warranting some type of institutionalization. The present choices are, basically, acute-care hospital or nursing home, but, as presently structured, these settings are too often inappropriate to satisfying needs of the terminal patient and family unit. An innovative, yet long-awaited alternative is the use of the hospice concept, which aims at anticipatory pain relief, as well as the psychological and comforting aspects of terminal care.

No extensive cost effectiveness study has yet been undertaken comparing hospital and hospice costs, taking into account the cost of planning and construction. In addition to assessing the feasibility of putting financial resources into these facilities, such a study would have implications for possible legislative changes regarding the 3-day hospitalization requirement for Medicare reimbursement. If indeed the cost of hospitalizing for 3 days before hospice care is greater than direct admittance to the hospice, it should not be classified as a posthospital extended-care benefit for Medicare purposes, but rather as a separate category of care facility that would need to be defined.

Because the development of hospices is a long-range goal and hospices may be able to serve only a portion of the target population, short-term goals should focus on ameliorating conditions for the terminally ill within existing hospitals and long-term care facilities. To do this, an extensive educational program should be organized in medical schools and in institutions, not only to teach methods of pain control and how to deal with dying patients, but also to enhance the concept of death as a natural process. Instruction dealing with psychological management should be an integral part of the training of physicians and nurses, as should continuing education of the same content for hospital staff.

As stated by Schonberg and Carr:[2b]

> Many university and teaching hospitals hold "death conferences" when a patient dies in order to determine if any additional efforts could have been expended in order to prolong the life of the individual patient. An appropriate parallel would be a "life conference" preceding death to determine what steps should be taken to assist the patient, family, and hospital personnel in managing the painful feeling of grief, guilt, depression, anxiety, and anger.

Of course, some professionals perhaps have a greater affinity than others for working with dying patients and their families. These people should be engaged as specialists in terminal care and be responsible for integrating efforts for a system of continuity of care. The result, it is hoped, would be an increased ability on the part of health professionals to recognize the unique and individual needs of these patients within an acute-care hospital. Although all hospital staff should be sensitized to problems in terminal care, the most effective management should probably take place in a separate ward where all staff would be specialists. Such a ward should be an appendage to the hospital in structure only and operate under a different routine and set of regulations that are more applicable to terminal care than to acute care. In short, the goal is to use existing facilities and expedite proper and appropriate care as a hospice within a hospital until such time that hospices are established in geographic areas where they are able to serve a large enough segment of the target population to be cost effective.

Because Medicare primarily covers people over age 65, a definite gap exists between reimbursement policies and the reality of occurrence of terminal illness, inclusive of all degenerative diseases. A large number of these diseases occur in people under 65, including children. The costs of care are so exorbitant that these illnesses are correctly categorized as "catastrophic," in regard to the devastating effect on patient and family, emotionally and financially. Legislative policy should parallel the need of a large segment of the population who are unable to meet the costs incurred by a long illness that ends in death. Just as patients with end-stage renal disease are eligible for reimbursement under Medicare, so should those afflicted with other catastrophic illnesses. The combined efforts of legislative change, educational programs, and realistic institutional changes emanating from the cultivation of medicine's art should aim at overcoming the defense mechanisms in the presence of death—denial, withdrawal, and avoidance—which manifest themselves in present institutional and professional practices.

NOTES

1. A. C. Weisman, "Psychosocial Considerations in Terminal Care," in *Psychosocial Aspects of Terminal Care* (New York: Columbia University Press, 1972), p. 163.

2. B. Schoenberg and A. C. Carr, "Educating the Health Professionals in the Psychosocial Care of the Terminally Ill," in *Psychosocial Aspects of Terminal Care* (New York: Columbia University Press, 1972), (a) p. 9, (b), p. 13.

3. M. Lerner, "When, Why, and Where People Die," in *The Dying Patient* (New York: Russell Sage Foundation, 1970), pp. 12-16.

4. D. Rabin and L. Rabin, "Consequences of Death for Physicians, Nurses, and Hospitals," in *The Dying Patient* (New York: Russell Sage Foundation, 1970), (a) p. 174, (b) p. 175, (c) p. 181.

5. R. J. Nelson, "Hospice: An Alternative Solution to the Problem of Caring for the Dying Patient, *Colloquy* (March 1974): 22-23.

6. H. S. Olin, "Failure and Fulfillment: Education in the Use of Psychoactive Drugs in the Dying Patient," in *Psychopharmacologic Agents for the Terminally Ill and Bereaved*. Foundation of Thanatology; distributed by Columbia University Press, New York, 1973.

7. B. G. Glaser and A. Strauss, *Awareness of Dying* (Chicago: Aldine Publication Company, 1965), p. 86.

8. A. Sheldon, C. P. Ryser, and M. J. Krant, "An Integrated Family Oriented Cancer Care Program: The Report of a Pilot Project in the Socio-emotional Management of Chronic Disease," *Journal of Chronic Disease* (April 1970): 22: 743-755.

9. G. L. Klerman, "Drugs and the Dying Patient," in *Psychopharmacologic Agents for the Terminally Ill and Bereaved*. Foundation of Thanatology; distributed by Columbia University Press, New York, 1973, p. 15.

10. T. H. Koff, "Social Rehearsal for Death and Dying." *Journal of Long-Term Care Administration* 3 (Summer 1975): 42-53.

11. D. Sudnow, "Dying in a public hospital," in *The Dying Patient* (New York: Russell Sage Foundation, 1970); (a) p. 191, (b) p. 194.

12. E. K. Ross, *On Death and Dying* (New York: The MacMillan Company, 1969).

13. J. Pollack, "Observations on the Economics of Illness," in *Proceedings of the Fourth National Symposium on Catastrophic Illness in the Seventies* (New York: Cancer Care, Inc. 1971), p. 26.

14. Cancer Care, Inc.: *The Impact, Cost and Consequences of Catastrophic Illness on Patients and Families* (New York, 1973), p. 54.

15. D. Maddison and B. Raphael, "The family of the dying patient," in *Psychosocial Aspects of Terminal Care* (New York: Columbia University Press, 1972), pp. 188-209.

16. C. Saunders, "Terminal Patient Care," *Geriatrics* 21 (December 1966): 70, 74.

17. Z. M. Cotter, "Institutional Care of the Terminally Ill," *Hospital Progress* 52: (June 1971): 52-48.

18. C. Saunders, *The Management of Terminal Illness* (London: Hospital Medicine Publications, Ltd., 1967), p. 23.

19. C. Saunders, "The patient's response to treatment," in *Proceedings of the Fourth National Symposium on Catastrophic Illness in the Seventies* (New York: Cancer Care, Inc., 1971); (a) p. 35, (b) p. 39.

20. R. C. Lamerton, "The Need for Hospices," *Nursing Times* (Jan. 23, 1975), p. 156.

21. S. Lack, "Death with Dignity at Home." *Washington Post* (Nov. 16, 1975).

Chapter 22

Future of Health Care for Elderly

This book has addressed various contemporary and historical problems of health care. As has been pointed out on numerous occasions, the size of the elderly population will increase substantially during the next 50 years, both in absolute numbers and as a percentage of the total population. As a result, we shall also see a substantial increase in the need and utilization of health care not only by the elderly as a group but also by the total population. Because an increasing share of the Gross National Product (GNP) will be used to provide health care for all, there will be considerable concern and interest in health care and in cost containment.

This final chapter explores a few areas that will impact on the health care delivery process and health care costs of the future. Some of these areas will improve the quality of health care and, indirectly, the quality of life. However, this can be accomplished only at a cost to the taxpayer.

REASONS WHY HEALTH CARE COSTS WILL KEEP RISING

Health care costs in the United States have reached a level of 9 percent of the GNP. However, we can anticipate a continuing rise in this percentage for a variety of reasons.

The United States has entered a service-oriented economy, and an increasing percentage of the GNP will be generated by services. Health care is clearly a service and will have at least its relative share of that percentage and most likely an increasing share. Eventually, health care will probably account for 12 percent of the GNP. This figure may not be reached before the turn of the century but possibly shortly thereafter.

This projected rise in health care costs is due not only to an increase in illness or more demand for current health care services. It also reflects (1) diagnostic, (2) evaluative, (3) therapeutic, and (4) curative procedures that have not yet been developed or are currently in the experimental stage. It is useful to review each of the four procedure areas in more detail to see how it adds to the total cost of health care.

Expansion of Diagnostic Procedures

Diagnostic procedures have been expanding at a rapid rate. Multiphasic screening, "CAT" scanners, and other procedures have made available to the physician a multitude of information for diagnostic purposes. The information available frequently exceeds the physician's experience, knowledge, and ability to make accurate diagnoses. However, the ability to generate information will go along with improvements in diagnostic abilities. In addition, the technical abilities of diagnostic equipment will clearly keep expanding.

The explosion in expensive, highly technical equipment has frequently been cited as one of the reasons for the rapidly escalating health care costs. To some extent this has been true, because equipment has been used to generate revenue instead of necessary diagnostic data. In other instances, the equipment was acquired without adequate demand, thus generating high per unit costs. Increased and enforced government regulation will reduce the number of instances where expensive and highly technical equipment is acquired by institutions for self-aggrandizement. The sharing of high cost, specialized equipment will become more common in the future.

Although the future will probably see a decline in outright waste through poor utilization of expensive equipment, the total cost of health care will undoubtedly keep rising. New technology will provide diagnostic data unheard of today. The beneficiaries will be those afflicted, but the costs will be borne by all.

Growth of Evaluative Procedures

The area of physical evaluation is still very much in its infancy. When one visits a physician for a physical examination, the physician usually provides only minimal information to the client. Only in case of a serious problem will the physician communicate the information to the client. If there are no problems, the results of the examination consist of a report that everything is normal.

It seems, however, that individuals are becoming more interested in using the various output measures of a physical evaluation to monitor their own condition. To some extent, an individual is capable of self-evaluation even now. Heart rate, temperature, and blood pressure are common measures one can monitor regularly. However, there are numerous other measures that require special assistance in the form of a physician or technician or a diagnostic device such as an x-ray, chemical laboratory test, etc.

Although the benefits of the detailed evaluations are by no means clear, it remains an area of considerable interest not only to the younger adults but also to the elderly. Since the evaluative procedures clearly fall into the category of preventive medicine, there will no doubt be considerable support for this trend. As a result, the cost of providing these procedures will be reimbursable under most third party arrangements, and this will add to health care costs.

Increase in Therapeutic Procedures

In the future rehabilitative therapy for mental and especially physical disabilities will be one of the most rapidly growing areas in health care. In the past the physically disabled patient has been relegated to a nonproductive, or at best partially productive citizen. But increasing interest and expansion of rehabilitative therapy will certainly change that. Although initially the resources of rehabilitative therapy will be devoted to younger persons who have longer productive life spans ahead of them, eventually, as the rehabilitative resource manpower increases, the elderly will reap the benefits of these therapies.

Again, the costs of providing these rehabilitative programs are high. At the top-notch institutions such as the Rehabilitation Institute of Chicago, a six-week rehabilitation program for patients with low back pain runs about $400 per day. These costs will be added to the costs of personal health care. What cannot be directly measured are the benefits society derives from having the rehabilitated lead a productive life.

Curative Procedures of the Future

Curative medicine, that area of medicine practiced by the majority of physicians, will clearly continue to expand. The largest growth area during the Seventies was heart by-pass surgery. The next 50 years will witness other developments that will increase the demand for those physicians trained in the needed specialties.

The increasing growth of the number of senior citizens will prompt a developing and increasing interest in the elderly. The geriatrician, now a rarity, will become as common as the pediatrician.

The field of medicine will continue to expand with new curative procedures and the addition of other specialties. The cost of supporting the expanded field will add to the cost of personal health care.

THE ELDERLY AS HEALTH CARE PROVIDERS

As the number of people over age 65 increases, there will simultaneously develop a potential shortage of skilled professionals to care for this group's health care needs. The result will be that organizations responsible for taking care of the elderly will increasingly turn to the younger elderly (such as those between 65 and 70) to rejoin the work force, possibly on a part-time basis, to care for the nonwell elderly in need of home care. This could well develop into a positive self-help movement whereby groups of elderly aid each other much along the lines of cooperative commercial developments of the past. Cooperative commercial developments, or "coops", have evolved in the past in response to a need that could not be satisfied by the private and government sectors. In response to this need people banded together to take care of their own needs in a cooperative but organized manner. There is no reason why this could not happen with the elderly.

As a side benefit the feeling of being needed and the importance of providing services that have real economic value could well boost the overall mental outlook of the elderly who now frequently feel shunted aside when they reach age 65.

CONCLUSIONS

The elderly as a group will grow in numbers and in strength, political, economic and otherwise. Their political strength will inspire more respect from and greater equality with the younger population. Economically, the elderly will be in better financial condition through improved government-financed retirement and health care programs. But they will continue to bear an increasing part of the economic burden through taxation (those with higher retirement incomes) and through economic participation (those able to participate in productive activities).

The elderly as a group will also change. At present, all those over 65 are grouped into one category. However, we may see the development of a single group of elderly starting at age 70. Alternatively, we may see two groups develop—the junior elderly consisting of those from 65 to 75, and the senior elderly consisting of those 75 and over.

If we want to obtain accurate health care statistics, there is a need to separate the elderly into two groups. Clearly, the current health care statistics for the elderly are too inexact because such a large age group displays widely varying health care needs.

The twenty-first century may be the beginning of a period when health care is widely available to all, without financial constraints. The cost to society will be substantial, but in a service-oriented society citizens must be willing to shoulder that burden. However, even as health care expenditures rise in excess of 12 percent of the GNP, we shall continue to hear the cry for cost containment.

Cost containment will continue to be of major concern to policy makers. However, cost containment will not be at the expense of the elderly. With their increased political and economic strength, they will be able to protect their interests and ensure that high quality health care will be available to all regardless of economic condition. We also shall see the passage of some form of catastrophic health insurance. Catastrophic health insurance will remove the costly nursing home care from the welfare (Medicaid) rolls and make nursing home care a right instead of a handout for those in need of it.

Index